Preventing Falls:

How to Develop Community-based
Fall Prevention Programs for Older Adults

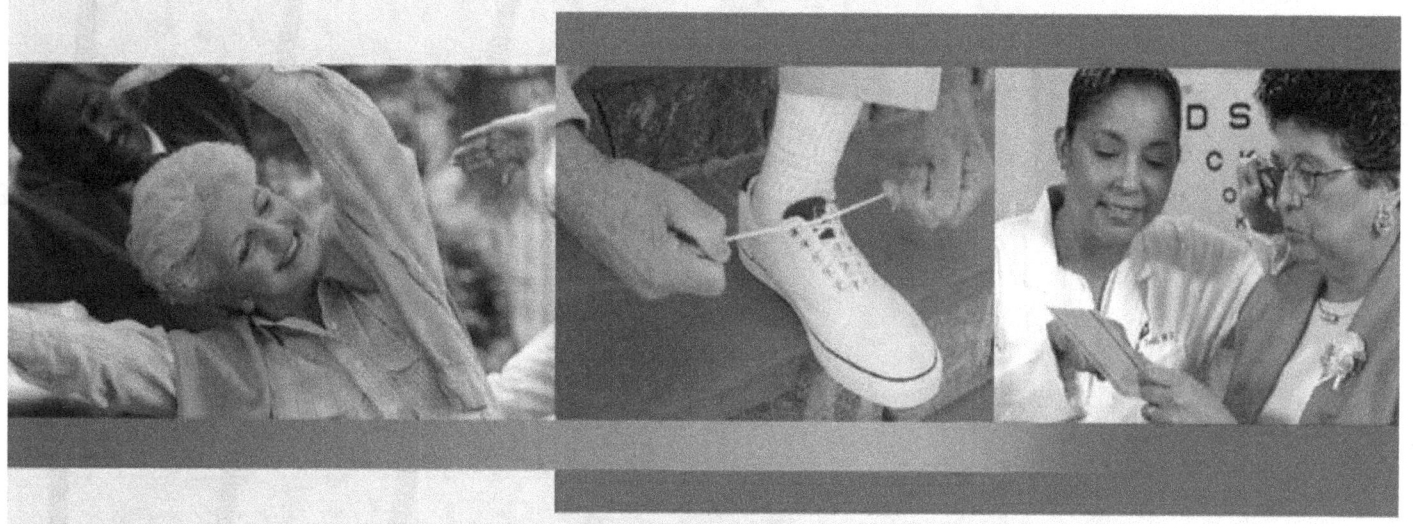

2008

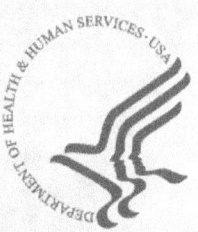

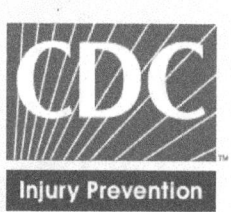

Preventing Falls:

How to Develop Community-based Fall Prevention Programs for Older Adults

National Center for Injury Prevention and Control

Atlanta, Georgia

2008

This document is a publication of the
National Center for Injury Prevention and Control
of the Centers for Disease Control and Prevention:

Centers for Disease Control and Prevention
Julie L. Gerberding, MD, MPH, Director

Coordinating Center for Environmental Health and Injury Prevention
Henry Falk, MD, MPH, Director

National Center for Injury Prevention and Control
Ileana Arias, PhD, Director

Division of Unintentional Injury Prevention
David Wallace, MSEH, Acting Director

Home and Recreation Injury Prevention Team
Michael Ballesteros, PhD, Team Leader

Acknowledgements

We acknowledge and appreciate the contributions of National Center for Injury Prevention and Control staff Judy Stevens, PhD, Michael Ballesteros, PhD, Michele Huitric, MPH, Amanda Tarkington, MC, Jane Mitchko, MEd, CHES, and Leslie Dorigo, MA. This project was assisted by Macro International Inc. Carol Freeman, BA, served as the Macro project director, Sally York, MN, RNC, and Mary E. Miller, MA, served as writer/editors and Lucinda Austin served as project assistant. Cover and text design by Monika Gullett, MA. We thank Thom Snyder, BA, MDiv, Ilene F. Silver, MPH, and Jane Mahoney, MD for their thorough review and valuable suggestions.

Suggested Citation: National Center for Injury Prevention and Control. Preventing Falls: How to Develop Community-based Fall Prevention Programs for Older Adults. Atlanta, GA: Centers for Disease Control and Prevention, 2008.

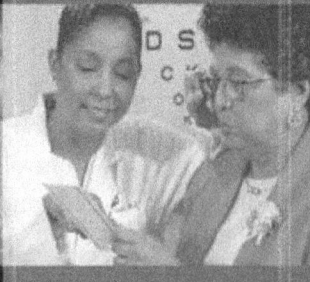

Contents

Chapter 1

Introduction

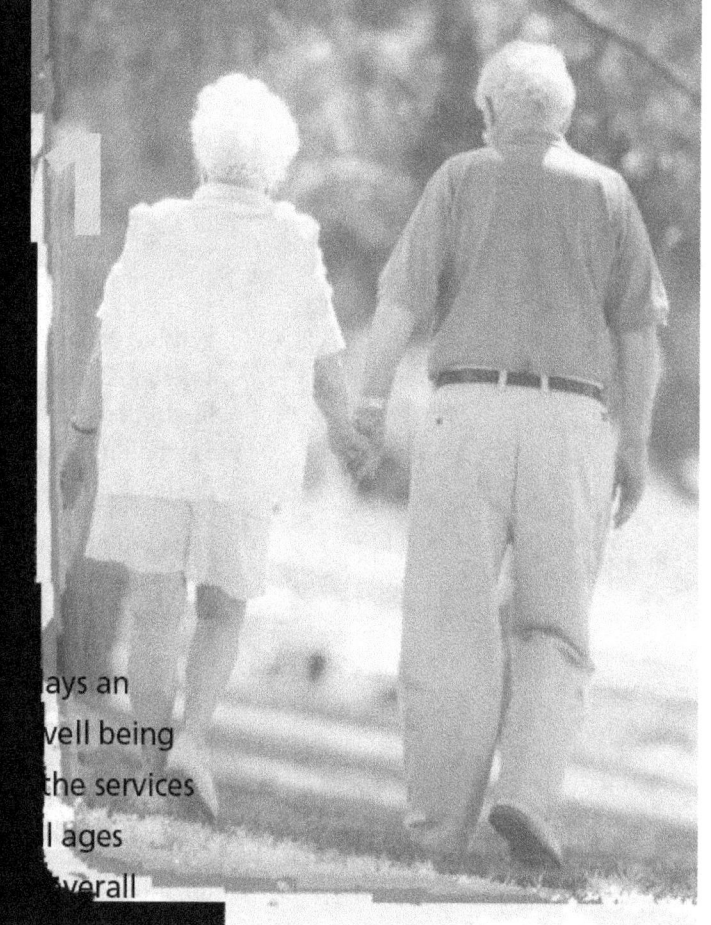

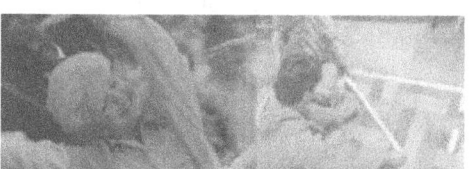

Your community-based organization (CBO) plays an important role in promoting the health and well being of the residents in your community. Many of the services provided by CBOs like yours help people of all ages maintain healthy lifestyles and improve their overall quality of life. Now, with the help of this new publication, *Preventing Falls: How to Develop Community-based Fall Prevention Programs for Older Adults*, your organization can reach out to the older members of your community and fulfill an increasingly important need for effective, community-based fall prevention programs.

Why fall prevention is important

Falls are a major threat to the health and independence of older adults, people aged 65 and older. Each year in the United States, nearly one-third of older adults experience a fall.

Falls can be devastating. About one out of ten falls among older adults result in a serious injury, such as a hip fracture or head injury, that requires hospitalization. In addition to the physical and emotional pain, many people need to spend at least a year recovering in a long-term care facility. Some never return to their homes.

Falls can be deadly. Falls are the leading cause of injury deaths among older adults. The rate of fall-related deaths among older adults in the United States has risen significantly over the past decade. In 2004, falls were responsible for 14,900 deaths.

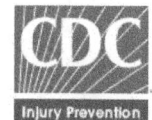

Falls are costly. Fall-related injuries among older adults, especially among older women, are associated with substantial economic costs. In 2000, direct medical costs for fatal and nonfatal fall injuries totaled $19 billion. As the number of older adults increases dramatically over the next few decades, so will the economic burden of falls.

Falls are preventable. The opportunity to help reduce falls among older adults has never been better. Today, there are effective fall prevention interventions that can be used in community settings. By offering effective fall prevention programs in our communities, we can reduce falls and help older adults live better, longer lives.

Understanding the risk factors for falls among older adults

Falls are not an inevitable consequence of aging, but falls do occur more often among older adults because fall risk factors increase with age and are usually associated with health and aging conditions. These risk factors include:

Biological risk factors

- Mobility problems due to muscle weakness or balance problems
- Chronic health conditions such as arthritis and stroke
- Vision changes and vision loss
- Loss of sensation in feet

Behavioral risk factors

- Inactivity
- Medication side effects and/or interactions
- Alcohol use

Environmental risk factors

- Home and environmental hazards (clutter, poor lighting, etc.)
- Incorrect size, type, or use of assistive devices (walkers, canes, crutches, etc.)
- Poorly designed public spaces

Usually two or more risk factors interact to cause a fall (such as poor balance and low vision, which can cause a trip and fall going up a single step). Home or environmental risk factors play a role in about half of all falls.

Understanding these risk factors is the first step to reducing older adult falls. Over the past two decades, researchers around the world have used descriptive studies to identify risk factors and randomized controlled trials to test fall interventions. The results of these studies show that reducing fall risk factors significantly reduces falls among community-dwelling older adults—those people living independently in the community.

Many older adults, as well as their family members and caregivers, are unaware of factors or behaviors that put them at risk of falling, and are also unaware of what actions they can take to reduce their risk. Fall risk factor assessment is rarely a part of an older adult's routine health care, even if they have had a fall or fall injury. All older adults should be encouraged to seek an individual fall risk assessment from their healthcare provider, especially older adults with a history of falls and/or with mobility or balance impairments who are at highest risk for falls.

A self-administered risk assessment form for older adults can be useful when the results are discussed with a healthcare provider who can help modify or manage identified risk factors.

Appendix A shows an example of a fall risk assessment developed by the Washington State Department of Health's Injury and Violence Prevention Program for individuals to use when discussing fall prevention with a healthcare professional.

Effective interventions can prevent older adult falls

Effective fall interventions reduce fall risk factors through either exercise alone or by combining exercise with other risk reduction approaches such as medication review and management, vision screening and correction, education, and safer living environments.

The Centers for Disease Control and Prevention (CDC) has reviewed and identified community-based fall prevention interventions that have strong scientific evidence of effectiveness.

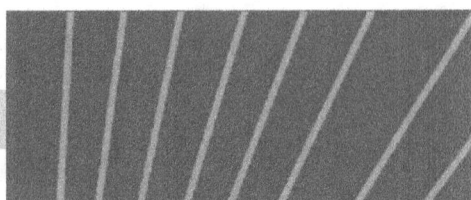

These interventions have been summarized and compiled in *Preventing Falls: What Works. A CDC Compendium of Effective Community-based Interventions from Around the World*, the companion publication to this document.

CDC would like to help CBOs move these proven fall interventions into communities to protect the health and independence of older adults.

Purpose of this guide

CDC developed this guide for communities and CBOs, so they can begin developing effective fall prevention programs. The main purpose of this guide is to:

- Define the key elements of what makes fall prevention programs effective
- Provide information to communities and CBOs on how to develop effective older adult fall prevention programs

This guide is intended to be used by CBO decisionmakers, program managers, and partners in organizations that serve independent living, community-dwelling older adults, such as:

- Public health departments
- Healthcare organizations that provide individual health care, individual or group community programs, and home-based services
- Hospital outpatient and community programs
- Senior and community centers
- Parks and recreation programs
- Emergency medical services
- Faith-based and parish nurse services and programs
- Home-based services (e.g., home health, meal-delivery services, chore services)
- Area Agencies on Aging

- Independent/retirement living, residential, and senior housing facilities/settings for older adults who live independently
- Nonprofit organizations that provide direct services to older adults
- Universities/community colleges that offer or work with community programs for community-dwelling older adults

Note: The interventions and programs in this guide are not designed for hospital inpatients, assisted living residents, Alzheimer's care programs and facilities, or nursing home residents, all of whom require programs and interventions that are specifically designed for their increased frailty and fall risk.

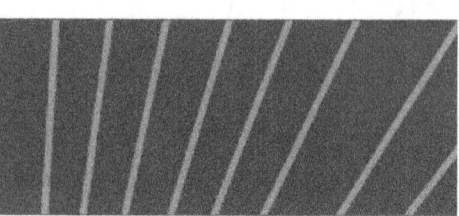

Notes:

Chapter 2

Planning an Effective
Fall Prevention Program

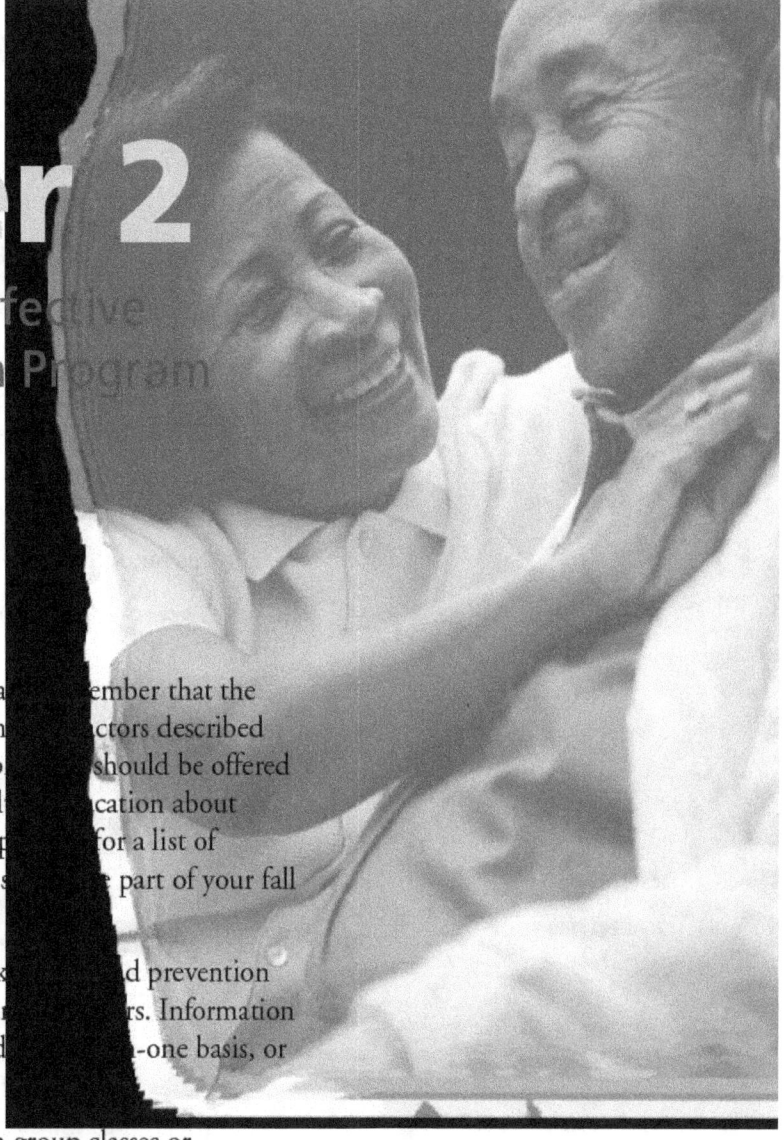

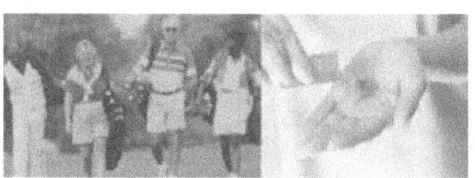

When planning your fall prevention progra... ...ember that the most effective programs address many of th... ...ctors described in Chapter 1. An effective fall prevention p... ...should be offered by trained healthcare professionals and incl... ...cation about falls and fall risk factors. (See the chart on p... ...for a list of professionals.) The main components that s... ...e part of your fall prevention program include the following:

- ☐ Education about older adult fall risk... ...d prevention strategies for older adults, families, a... ...rs. Information can be communicated on an individ... ...-one basis, or in a group setting.

- ☐ Exercise that can be offered through group classes or individually. Exercise programs can be offered in a community setting, at home with supervision, or in a program that combines group classes or one-on-one training with home-based exercise. Appropriate types of exercises that effectively reduce falls in older adults include:

  - Tai Chi
  - Strengthening exercises combined with balance training
  - Balance exercises

- ☐ Medication review by a pharmacist or healthcare professional, with medication adjusted or modified by a physician or nurse practitioner.
- ☐ Vision assessment and vision correction by an optometrist or ophthalmologist.
- ☐ Home safety assessment including home modifications as needed.

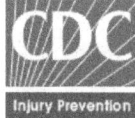

These building blocks of an effective fall prevention program are discussed in more detail in Chapter 5, but keep them in mind during the planning process for your program.

Key steps in developing a fall prevention program

Follow this nine-step process in planning your fall prevention program.

Step 1. Assess your community's needs.
Before deciding what type of fall prevention program to develop, use the following checklist to assess your community's needs and identify appropriate resources:

- ☐ What are the fall prevention program needs in your community?
- ☐ What related programs or services are currently being offered by other organizations?
- ☐ What are your organization's current and future goals and resources for providing services to independent older adults in your community?
- ☐ How much support for starting a fall prevention program is there at all levels of your organization—from the board and director, to the staff, volunteers, and older adult clients?
- ☐ What community resources exist that could provide services to address older adult fall risk factors?
- ☐ What community resources and organizations are potential partners?

Step 2. Establish your program's purpose, goals, and objectives.
Develop a purpose statement and determine the goals and objectives of your program. Ask questions such as, "Why are we developing this program?" and "What do we hope to accomplish both short term and long term?" Your purpose and goals should be specific, realistic, and clearly stated. Goals should be quantitative with objectives that can be easily measured. Think of the goal as a destination and the objectives as methods of getting you to your goal. With a clear set of objectives, you can easily measure the success of your program during the evaluation phase. With a solid purpose, concrete goals, and action-oriented objectives, you can build an effective fall prevention program for older adults.

Step 3. Determine what risk factors your program will address.
There are two types of effective fall prevention programs: single intervention and multifaceted intervention programs:

☐ *Single intervention programs*

Exercise is the only intervention that by itself reduces falls among older adults. Many organizations have developed group and/or individualized exercise programs for older adults that improve strength and balance. You can develop an exercise program by using the information in this guide and working with trained professionals in your community. See Chapter 5 on page 21 for examples of effective exercise programs and related resources.

☐ *Multifaceted intervention programs*

A multifaceted intervention combines exercise with other intervention components to reduce fall risk factors. Such a program might include exercise, vision assessment, and fall prevention education. To create the most effective fall prevention program, begin with exercise and incorporate at least one other intervention component.

Step 4. Collaborate with partners to address additional risk factors. Partnering with other organizations can help you develop a more comprehensive and effective fall prevention program. Chapter 3 will provide more detail on how to identify and work with fall prevention partners.

Step 5. Decide who will implement the various program components. The following chart shows which healthcare providers and other professionals can deliver each type of intervention.

9

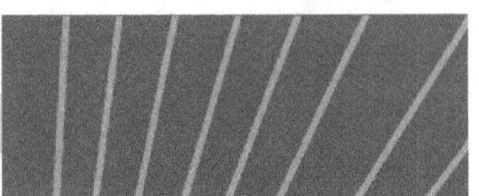

Who Can Deliver Fall Prevention Program Components?											
Program components	Physician	Optometrist	Nurse Practitioner/PA	Pharmacist	Registered Nurse	Physical Therapist	Occupational Therapist	Social Worker	Certified Exercise Instructor	Exercise Sci/Phys Ed Degree	Tai Chi Instructor
Education											
Group			✓		✓	✓	✓	✓*	✓*	✓*	✓*
Individual			✓	✓	✓	✓	✓	✓*	✓*	✓*	✓*
Assessment											
Gait	✓*		✓*			✓					
Balance; simple	✓*		✓*		✓*	✓	✓*		✓*	✓*	✓*
Balance; in-depth	✓*		✓*		✓*	✓	✓*				
Strength	✓*		✓*		✓*	✓	✓*		✓*	✓*	✓*
Exercise											
1:1 balance alone						✓	✓		✓*	✓*	✓*
1:1 strength with balance training						✓	✓		✓	✓*	
Group class						✓*	✓		✓	✓*	✓
Individualized exercise/PT			✓		✓	✓	✓		✓		✓
Tai Chi									✓*	✓*	✓
Medication											
Medication review			✓	✓	✓*						
Medication management	✓										
Vision											
Basic assessment	✓	✓	✓*		✓*						
Detailed assessment	✓										
Vision correction	✓	✓									
Home Safety											
Assessment			✓*		✓*	✓*	✓	✓*			
Basic modification**					✓	✓	✓	✓*			
Skilled modification**							✓				
Other											
Assistive device training						✓	✓				

* Additional specialized education and training required
** Basic modification includes clutter/throw rug removal, rearrange furniture; skilled modification includes grab bars, ramps, electrical work.

Note: Partnerships may facilitate delivering multifaceted programs in community settings.

Step 6. Find a location to conduct the program. When considering what type of program to develop, consider the types of places where a program can be held. The following chart provides suggestions for each type of fall prevention component.

Where to Conduct Fall Prevention Program Components								
Program components	Home	Physician Office	Hospital/Clinic (outpatient)	PT Facility	Pharmacy	Senior/Community Rec Center	Gym/Fitness Center/ Rec Center	Senior Housing Facility
Education								
Group			✓			✓	✓	✓
Individual	✓	✓	✓	✓	✓	✓	✓	✓
Assessment								
Gait	✓	✓	✓	✓		✓	✓	✓
Balance; simple	✓	✓	✓	✓		✓	✓	✓
Balance; in-depth	✓	✓	✓	✓		✓	✓	✓
Strength	✓	✓	✓	✓		✓	✓	✓
Exercise								
1:1 balance alone	✓		✓	✓		✓	✓	✓
1:1 strength with balance training	✓		✓	✓		✓	✓	✓
Group class						✓	✓	✓
Individualized exercise/PT	✓		✓	✓		✓	✓	✓
Tai Chi						✓	✓	✓
Medication								
Medication review	✓	✓	✓		✓	✓	✓	✓
Medication management		✓	✓		✓			
Vision								
Basic assessment	✓	✓	✓			✓		✓
Detailed assessment		✓	✓					
Vision correction		✓	✓					
Home Safety								
Assessment	✓							✓
Basic modification**	✓							✓
Skilled modification**	✓							✓
Other								
Assistive device training	✓	✓	✓	✓		✓	✓	✓

** Basic modification includes clutter/throw rug removal, rearrange furniture; skilled modification includes grab bars, ramps, electrical work.

Note: Partnerships may facilitate delivering multifaceted programs in community settings.

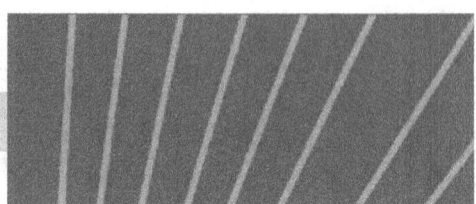

Step 7. Evaluate your program. Evaluation helps determine whether a program is appropriate and effective. The results of the evaluation will guide you in maintaining or modifying any aspects of the program and tell you if the program is worth continuing. Chapter 6 will help you develop evaluation strategies to document your program's effectiveness.

Step 8. Promote your program. Making the community aware of your fall prevention program is crucial to its success. No matter the size of your outreach effort, Chapter 7 will help you in developing a campaign to publicize your program and provide you with tips on working with your local media.

Step 9. Sustain your program. To sustain your program, you will need to review and make modifications. This means keeping sight of your goals and maintaining momentum in building collaborations, advocating for support, and seeking new sources of funding. Chapter 8 will help guide you through this process.

Chapter

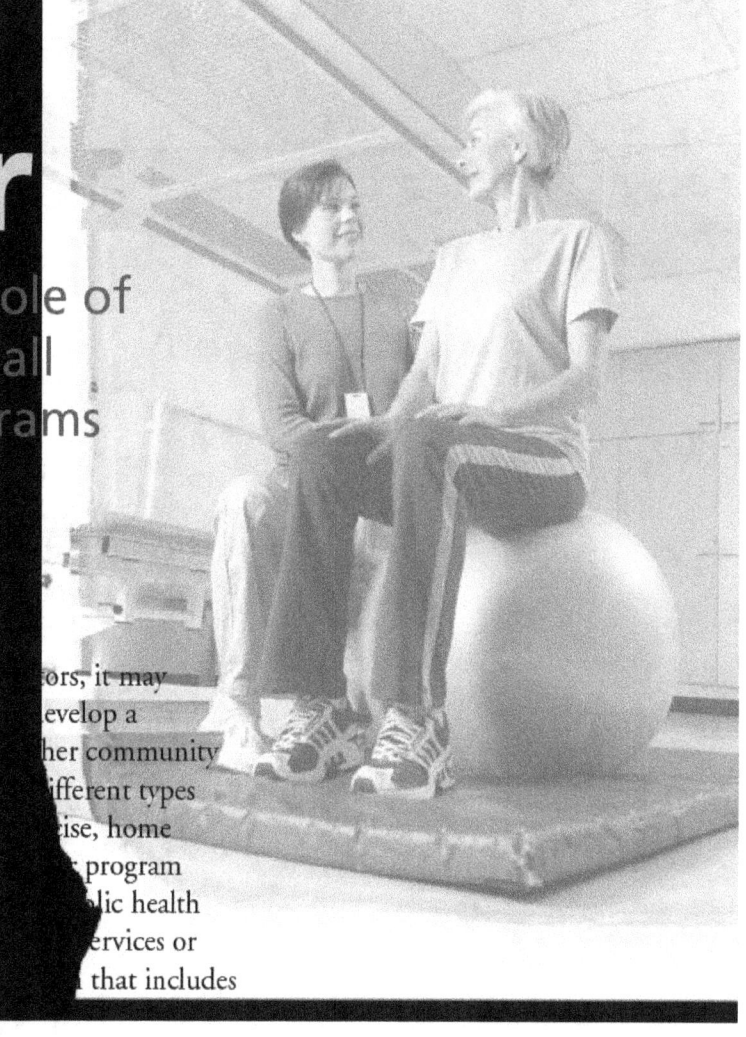

The Important Role of Partnerships in Fall Prevention Programs

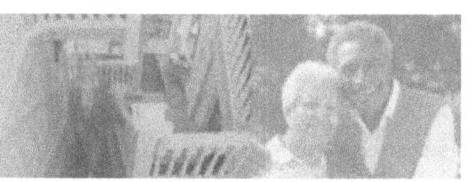

Because falls are the result of multiple fall risk factors, it may be difficult for your organization, on its own, to develop a comprehensive program. By collaborating with other community organizations and professionals that specialize in different types of services for older adults, such as healthcare, exercise, home safety assessment, and education, you can make your program more comprehensive and effective. For example, a public health or healthcare organization may partner with social services or parks and recreation organization to create a program that includes exercise and fall prevention education.

Collaborating with other CBOs can provide additional resources, outreach channels, or referral sources for your program. Because of its many benefits, collaboration can be essential in developing your program.

How to develop partnerships

- ☐ **Assess your current situation.** Planning your prevention program involves a careful analysis of your organizational resources and needs, including staff, funding, facilities, technology, and expertise. This information clarifies when a potential partnership with another organization can support your program goals.

- ☐ **Identify potential partners.** Partnerships should be mutually beneficial. Identify organizations that share your mission of improving health and safety for older adults or that have a vested interest in reducing falls among older adults. Determine how a collaboration will mutually support short- and long-term goals.

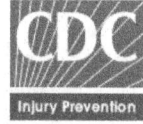

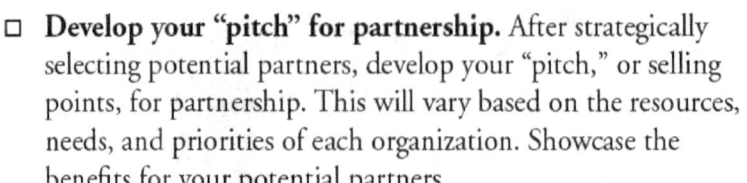

☐ **Develop your "pitch" for partnership.** After strategically selecting potential partners, develop your "pitch," or selling points, for partnership. This will vary based on the resources, needs, and priorities of each organization. Showcase the benefits for your potential partners.

☐ **Create your messages and materials.** Develop message points—short, concise statements that reflect your main messages. These are useful for internal and external communications, as well as for presentations to partners.

For these messages:

- Develop themes or adapt materials that will engage your potential partners.
- Produce materials (computer-generated presentations, flyers, etc.) that will effectively convey your messages.
- Pretest your materials among potential partners.
- Develop a method for tracking partnerships and other outreach efforts.

☐ **Make contact.** Whenever possible, deliver your partnership proposal in person. Consider bringing at least one other person, because different communication styles and demeanors can influence an encounter. Sharing the workload and presentation delivery reduces the pressure of thinking on your feet. However, make sure that your team speaks with one voice, based on the messages you develop. Delivering mixed messages creates confusion and weakens your credibility.

☐ **Seal the deal.** Being credible and offering incentives are important, but these may not be enough to seal the deal. Use your passion to make potential partners believe they should be involved.

- Describe how your programs and services can make a difference.
- Share information about the burden of falls and fall injuries.
- Underscore how your community will benefit from your efforts and how others are getting involved.

- Remind potential partners of their strengths and how even seemingly small contributions can help prevent injury and death.
- Confirm how the proposed partnership is mutually beneficial.
- Be specific about what you are asking them to contribute and do.

How to maintain partnerships

Relationships need to be maintained. While commitment is important, so is continuing to review your resources, needs, and expectations as the program evolves. Involving local organizations will be an ongoing effort, so remember to engage as many facets of your community as you can, including:

- Hospitals and healthcare centers
- Local and state government officials and offices
- Faith-based organizations
- Civic organizations
- Senior citizen groups
- Commercial establishments serving older adults
- Clubs that may have a large older-adult membership (such as the Veterans of Foreign Wars)
- Universities or colleges that offer academic programs or services for older adults

Never forget the power of the phrase "thank you." Acknowledge partnership agreements promptly. Look for creative ways to convey your gratitude to partners often and thank them publicly. See Appendix B for an inventory form that can be useful for identifying community resources and potential program partners.

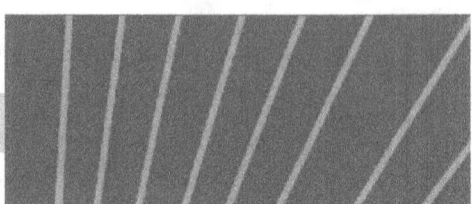

Partnership web resources

The National Council on Aging's Partnering to Promote Healthy Aging: Creative Best Practice Community Partnerships
www.healthyagingprograms.org/content.asp?sectionid=92&ElementID=160

Falls Free: A National Falls Prevention Action Plan
www.healthyagingprograms.org/content.asp?sectionid=98

California Blueprint For Falls Prevention
www.archstone.org/publications2292/publications_show.htm?doc_id=246660

Queensland, Australia Statewide Action Plan: Falls Prevention in Older People 2002-2006
www.health.qld.gov.au/phs/Documents/shpu/13693.pdf

WA State Dept. of Health Report - Falls Among Older Adults: Strategies for Prevention
www.doh.wa.gov/hsqa/emstrauma/injury/pubs/FallsAmongOlderAdults.pdf

Health care & public health partnerships
repositories.cdlib.org/cgi/viewcontent.cgi?article=1003&context=iha

Community Toolbox for Public Health Partnerships
ctb.ku.edu/WST/initiatives_show.jsp?initiative_id=44

Partnership self-assessment tool
www.cacsh.org/psat.html

Chapter 4

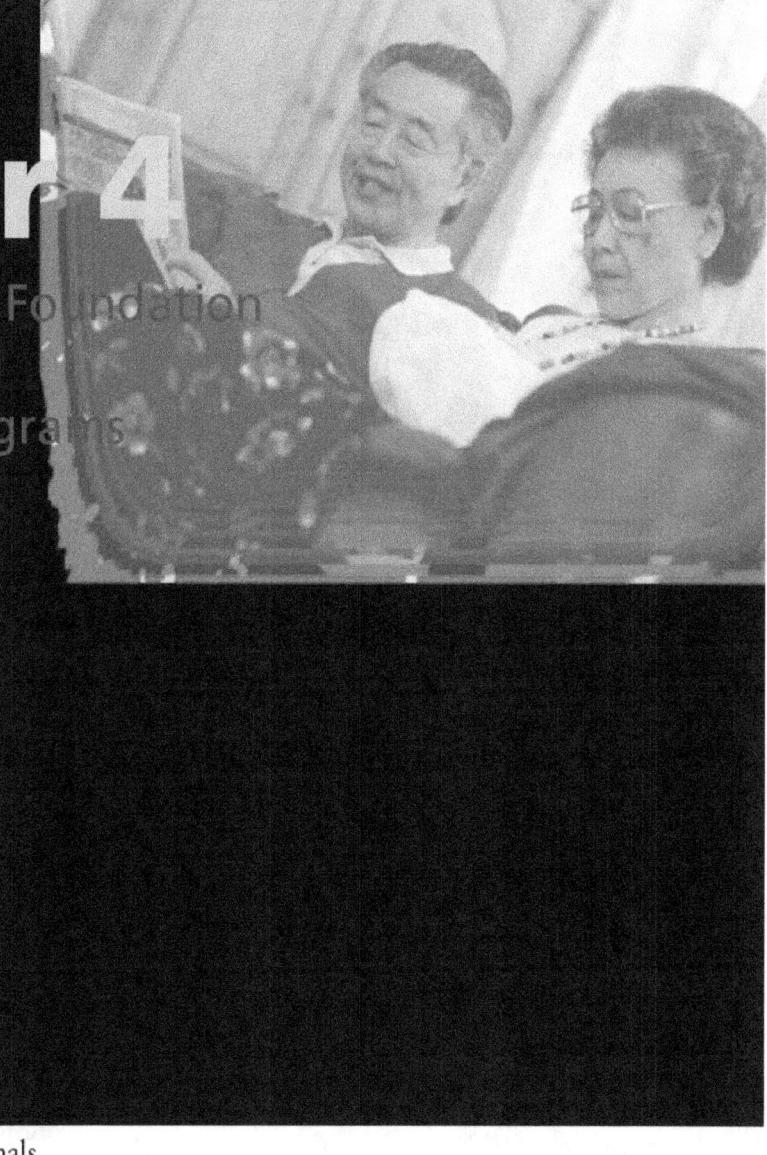

Education: The Foundation of Effective Fall Prevention Programs

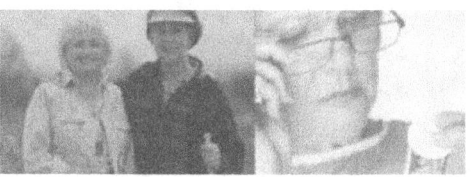

Increasing awareness about fall risk factors [and] risk is crucial in helping older adults, their [families and] service providers to effectively prevent falls.

There are two types of audiences for fall pr[evention:] professionals who will implement the fall p[rograms and] older adults and their caregivers.

People in your community who are qualifie[d to provide] professional fall prevention education sessi[ons include:]

- Healthcare professionals
- Public health professionals
- Senior service providers
- Emergency medical service professionals

Provider education

Provider education is necessary to inform healthcare and senior service providers about the current state of knowledge in fall prevention for older adults. Key aspects of professional education include:

- National, state, and county data on fatal and nonfatal fall injuries and healthcare costs. National and some state data are available from CDC's National Center for Injury Prevention and Control. Additional state and county data may be available from health departments, local emergency services, and fire departments. Data on cost of falls may be available from local hospitals.

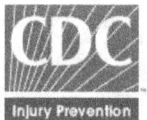

- Information about fall risk factors among older adults (see the web resources at the end of this chapter).
- Information about effective fall prevention interventions (see the web resources at the end of this chapter and the *Compendium*).
- Tools and resources to train professional staff to deliver fall prevention information tailored to their audience (see the web resources at the end of each chapter and the *Compendium*).

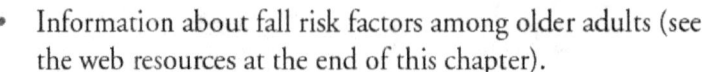

Fall Intervention Studies that Include Education

Stay Active, Stay Safe (Barnett, et al.)
The Otago Exercise Program (Campbell, et al., Robertson, et al.)
Tai Chi: Moving for Better Balance (Li, et al.)
Australian Group Exercise Program (Lord, et al.)
Simplified Tai Chi (Wolf, et al.)
Home Visits by an Occupational Therapist (Cumming, et al.)
Falls-HIT (Home Intervention Team) Program (Nikolaus, et al.)
Stepping On (Clemson, et al.)
PROFET (Prevention of Falls in the Elderly Trial) (Close, et al.)
The NoFalls Intervention (Day, et al.)
The SAFE Health Behavior and Exercise Intervention (Hornbrook, et al.)
Yale FICSIT (Frailty and Injuries: Cooperative Studies of Intervention Techniques) (Tinetti, et al.)
A Multifactorial Program (Wagner, et al.)

For more details, refer to the companion publication, Preventing Falls: What Works. A CDC Compendium of Effective Community-based Interventions from Around the World

Public education

Public education includes communicating the importance of fall prevention to the general public and directly informing older adults how to maintain a healthy lifestyle that reduces the risk of falls. When promoting your fall prevention program, you will also be creating awareness for the necessity of fall prevention in your community. You can find more information in Chapter 7 about promoting fall prevention and your fall prevention program.

Educating older adults about individual risks and methods of prevention is an important building block of every fall prevention program. More information on educating older adults about the risk of falls and fall prevention activities will follow in the next chapter.

Education web resources

CDC's "What You Can Do To Prevent Falls" and "Home Safety Checklist" brochures for older adults
www.cdc.gov/ncipc/duip/fallsmaterials.htm

CDC Falls Prevention page
www.cdc.gov/ncipc/duip/preventadultfalls.htm

Center of Excellence for Fall Prevention
www.stopfalls.org

National Institute on Aging, AgePage: Preventing Falls and Fractures
www.niapublications.org/agepages/PDFs/preventing_Falls_and_Fractures.pdf

The American Geriatrics Society Guideline for the Prevention of Falls in Older Persons
www.americangeriatrics.org/products/positionpapers/abstract.shtml

Center for Healthy Aging Falls Free Electronic News
www.healthyagingprograms.org

California Blueprint for Falls Prevention
www.archstone.org/publications2292/publications_show.htm?doc_id=246660

National Safety Council
www.nsc.org/issues/fallstop.htm

"Getting Up From a Fall" handout from the American Academy of Orthopaedic Surgeons
orthoinfo.aaos.org/topic.cfm?topic=A00098

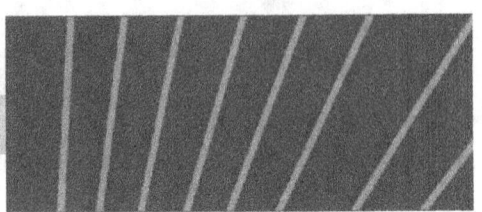

Notes:

Chapter 5

The 5 Building Blocks of Effective Community-based Fall Prevention Programs

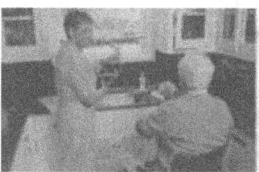 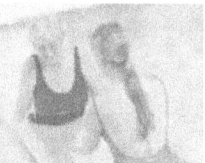

The most effective fall prevention programs factors described in Chapter 1. Based on y start your program using one building block effectiveness by adding more blocks over ti

The five main building blocks of an effective prevention program are:

☐ **Education** about falls and fall risk fa

☐ **Exercises** that improve mobility, stre
and that are taught by trained, natio
instructors or physical therapists. Ex

- Tai Chi
- Individualized exercise sessions
- Group exercise classes
- Home exercise programs with supervision until the older adult can exercise independently

☐ **Medication review** to identify side effects or drug interactions that may contribute to falls. The reviews should be conducted by pharmacists or healthcare providers. Medication management—adjustments to or changes in medications—should be provided by physicians.

☐ **Vision exams** by trained healthcare professionals with vision correction by an optometrist or ophthalmologist.

☐ **Home safety assessment and home modification** by occupational therapists or other healthcare professionals with specialized training, to identify and modify home hazards that can increase older adults' risk of falling.

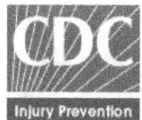

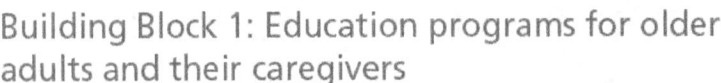

Building Block 1: Education programs for older adults and their caregivers

When developing a fall prevention program, it is important to include an educational component. While education alone has not proven to effectively reduce falls among older adults, it is typically combined with one of the other building blocks. Education for older adults and their caregivers can be delivered to individuals or to groups. Individual education sessions may work better for people who are hearing or vision impaired or have special needs. Sessions should be tailored to the attention span and cognitive ability of older adults. Visual aids such as brochures, fact sheets, and checklists will help facilitate the education session.

Group sessions provide the benefits of social interactions. Informal group discussions that include sharing personal experiences may reduce anxiety and increase motivation to adopt new behaviors. Group teaching saves time and helps spread the information more quickly to more people.

Tips for developing an effective education component

- ☐ Education should be delivered by trained professionals.
- ☐ Education should include problem solving and goal setting on the part of the learner.
- ☐ The length of the education session should depend on the individual characteristics of the older adult, such as concentration, hearing or visual impairment, etc.
- ☐ Group vs. individual education may be determined based on which other bulding block is being offered in combination.
- ☐ Visual aids are valuable tools in increasing comprehension.
- ☐ Materials should be designed with a high contrast background and large lettering.
- ☐ Materials should reflect literacy levels and be culturally appropriate.
- ☐ Presentations and materials should not contain abbreviations and jargon.
- ☐ Education is most effective when offered on an ongoing basis.

22

There is a wealth of educational materials available on the Internet. You can find visual aids, including posters, videos and presentations, brochures, and checklists, or you can develop your own materials. See Appendices C and D for an example of a brochure and a presentation. A set of fall prevention posters is also available through the CDC website listed below. Use the following websites for additional education materials.

Education web resources

CDC's "What You Can Do To Prevent Falls" and "Home Safety Checklist" brochures for older adults
www.cdc.gov/ncipc/pub-res/toolkit/brochures.htm

CDC Falls Prevention page
www.cdc.gov/ncipc/duip/preventadultfalls.htm

Center of Excellence for Fall Prevention
www.stopfalls.org

National Institute on Aging, AgePage: Preventing Falls and Fractures
www.niapublications.org/agepages/PDFs/preventing_Falls_and_Fractures.pdf

The American Geriatrics Society Guideline for the Prevention of Falls in Older Persons
www.americangeriatrics.org/products/positionpapers/abstract.shtml

Center for Healthy Aging Falls Free Electronic News
www.healthyagingprograms.org

California Blueprint for Falls Prevention
www.archstone.org/publications2292/publications_show.htm?doc_id=246660

American Academy of Orthopaedic Surgeons
orthoinfo.aaos.org/menus/safety.cfm

National Safety Council
www.nsc.org/issues/fallstop.htm

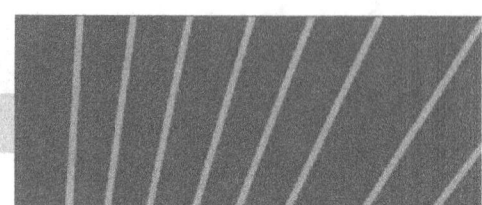

Building Block 2: Progressive exercise programs to improve mobility, strength, and balance

Among older adults, strength and balance exercises, such as Tai Chi, can reduce falls by improving mobility, strength, and balance. These programs focus on exercises that are specifically designed or adapted for older adults.

Tips for developing an effective exercise component

☐ To be safe and effective, older adult exercise programs (one-on-one or group classes) must be taught by one or more of the following professionals:

- Nationally certified fitness/exercise instructors with specialized training in working with older adults. Because exercise instructors are not licensed, having a national certification or accreditation is the minimum qualification requirement for teaching fall prevention exercise programs to older adults.

- Exercise science/physiology professionals with a bachelor's degree or master's degree in this field.

- Physical therapists.

- Occupational therapists.

- Recreational therapists with a bachelor's or master's degree.

- Tai Chi instructors, masters or grand masters, who have completed a Tai Chi course taught by a Tai Chi master or grand master, have a national certification in older adult physical activity, and have experience in teaching exercise to older adults.

- Physical, occupational, and recreational therapy assistants who are under the direct supervision of a physical, occupational, or recreational therapist.

Fall Intervention Studies that Include Exercise

Stay Active, Stay Safe (Barnett, et al.)
The Otago Exercise Program (Campbell, et al., Robertson, et al.)
Tai Chi: Moving for Better Balance (Li, et al.)
Australian Group Exercise Program (Lord, et al.)
Veterans Affair Group Exercise Program (Rubinstein, et al.)
Simplified Tai Chi (Wolf, et al.)
Home Visits by an Occupational Therapist (Cumming, et al.)
Falls-HIT (Home Intervention Team) Program (Nikolaus, et al.)
Stepping On (Clemson, et al.)
The NoFalls Intervention (Day, et al.)
The SAFE Health Behavior and Exercise Intervention (Hornbrook, et al.)
Yale FICSIT (Frailty and Injuries: Cooperative Studies of Intervention Techniques) (Tinetti, et al.)
A Multifactorial Program (Wagner, et al.)

For more details, refer to the companion publication, Preventing Falls: What Works. A CDC Compendium of Effective Community-based Interventions from Around the World

24

PROGRAMS IN ACTION

Stay Active and Independent for Life (SAIL):
A strength and balance fitness class for adults 65+

The SAIL program combines health information with exercises specifically designed to safely and easily improve endurance, strength, and balance in adults aged 65 and older. The program was researched and developed as a community-based fall prevention program by the Washington State Department of Health.

The SAIL program helps older adults to stay active and independent. It helps to prevent falls, through group exercise classes that meet for 1 hour, three times a week. The classes are held at community sites, such as senior centers, parks and recreation facilities, and community fitness centers that often work in partnership with community healthcare and senior service organizations to offer the program. Classes are led by certified fitness instructors who have attended the 2-day SAIL Instructor Training Program, which was designed by physical therapists and a registered nurse.

The program name and its key messages were developed through older adult focus groups to emphasize a specific description of the program and its positive benefits:

- "It works…you'll be stronger, have better balance, feel better, and this will help you stay independent, active, and prevent falls."
- "It's safe…the instructors are experienced and skilled, and exercises have been tested with seniors."
- "It's fun…you'll meet other seniors and make new friends."

The SAIL class exercises are designed to be done either sitting or standing, and at individually adjustable paces. The class includes aerobic and balance exercises, strength training with wrist and ankle weights, and flexibility exercises. The class participants also receive brief "Fitness Checks" when they start the classes for measuring progress and improvement after they start the classes. These measurements of walking speed and arm and leg strength, are repeated every 3 to 6 months throughout the year, enabling class participants to monitor their individual progress. In addition to the exercises, health information is included in the classes, which addresses topics such as exercising safely, medication and home safety, and footwear and foot care. The education information is provided in a booklet published by the Washington State Department of Health: "Stay Active and Independent for Life: An Information Guide for Adults 65+." All class participants receive a free copy of the booklet.

For more information contact:

www.cdc.gov/ncipc/profiles/core_state/wa/default.htm or
www.doh.wa.gov/hsqa/emstrauma/injury/pubs/default.htm#seniorfalls

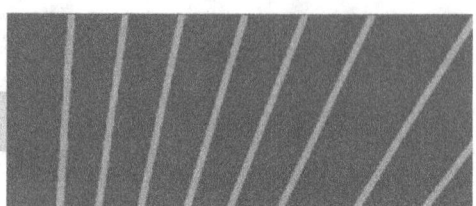

☐ All professionals who teach exercise to older adults must have a current CPR/AED certification.

☐ To be effective in reducing falls, exercises must be performed at least twice weekly on an ongoing basis and progress in difficulty throughout the program.

☐ Ideally, the exercise classes should be offered on an ongoing basis for long-term attendance. Short-term programs that have a set number of sessions should provide written instructions so participants can continue to do the exercises at home.

☐ Participants should be taught the exercises under the direct supervision of a trained exercise instructor or physical or occupational therapist, either in one-on-one home sessions or in group sessions, before performing them independently at home.

☐ Evaluate how the program instructor delivers the exercise program. Use process evaluation methods to ensure that the exercises are being taught properly and consistently. Also, obtain feedback from the program participants.

☐ Base program content on current published materials specifically developed for older adults by exercise science, physical therapy, or Tai Chi professionals.

☐ Assess older adults' strength, balance, and fitness at the beginning and end of each new exercise program.

☐ Limit the number of participants in group classes to no more than 15 to allow the instructor the ability to closely observe and supervise participants during the class session.

The National Council on Aging's Center for Healthy Aging has developed a detailed checklist for fall prevention programs in Evidence-based Healthy Aging Programming: Tools and Checklists at healthyagingprograms.org/content.asp?sectionid=32&ElementID=439

Appendix E provides examples of strengthening and balance exercises from the Stay Safe Stay Active Daily Exercise Program. Additional exercise examples can be found in the *Preventing Falls: What Works. A CDC Compendium of Effective Community-based Interventions from Around the World.*

Exercise program web resources

CDC Physical Activity Resources
www.cdc.gov/nccdphp/dnpa/physical

**National Council on Aging: Center for Healthy Aging, 2005.
Evidence-based Healthy Aging Programming: Tools
and Checklists**
www.healthyagingprograms.org

**International Curriculum Guidelines for Preparing Physical
Activity Instructors of Older Adults**
www.seniorfitness.net/international_curriculum_guidelines_for_
preparing_physical_activity_instructors_of_older_adults.htm

**Growing Stronger: Strength Training for Older Adults—a web
based strength training exercise program**
www.cdc.gov/nccdphp/dnpa/physical/growing_stronger

**National Institutes of Health: NIH Publication No. 01-4256, 2001
Exercise: A Guide from the National Institute on Aging**
www.nia.nih.gov/HealthInformation/Publications/ExerciseGuide

**National Council on Aging: Center for Healthy Aging,
Issue Brief #2, Winter 2004 Designing Safe and Effective
Physical Activity Programs**
www.healthyagingprograms.com/resources/IssueBrief_
PhysicalActivity.pdf

**National Council on Aging: Center for Healthy Aging,
Issue Brief #4, Fall 2005 Keeping Current on Research and
Practice in Physical Activity for Older Adults**
www.healthyagingprograms.com/resources/IssueBrief_
KeepCurrentPA.pdf

**National Council on Aging: Center for Healthy Aging, Moving
Ahead: Strategies and Tools to Plan, Conduct and Maintain
Effective Community-based Physical Activity Programs for
Older Adults**
www.healthyagingprograms.com/resources/PRC-HAN_conference_
monograph.pdf

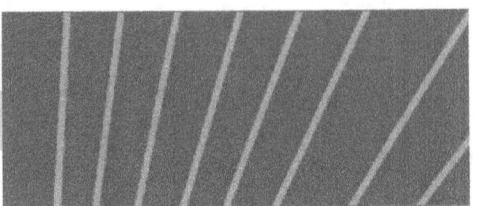

American College of Sports Medicine's Physical Activity Guidelines for adults over age 65
www.acsm.org/AM/Template.cfm?Section=Home_Page&
TEMPLATE=/CM/HTMLDisplay.cfm&CONTENTID=
7764#Over_65_or_50_64

Human Kinetics' Senior Fitness Test Manual and Software: manual and software for testing and tracking functional fitness measures in older adults
www.humankinetics.com/products/showproduct.cfm?isbn=
9780736033589

American Council on Exercise and AARP Fitness Resources
www.aarpfitness.com

Exercise and Older Adults
nihseniorhealth.gov/exercise/toc.html

References

Berg K. Balance and its measure in the elderly: A review. *Physiother*, Canada. 1989:41;240-246.

Chang JT, Morton SC, Rubenstein LZ, et al. Interventions for the prevention of falls in older adults: Systematic review and meta-analysis of randomized clinical trials. *Br Med Journal*. 2004:328;680-683.

Cotton, RT. *Exercise for older adults: American Council on Exercise's guide for fitness professionals.* Human Kinetics: Champaign, IL;1998.

Dunkin, A. *All you need to know about back pain.* Arthritis Foundation: Atlanta, GA;2002.

Gillespie LD, Gillespie WJ, Robertson MC, Lamb SE, Cumming RG, Rowe BH. Interventions for preventing falls in elderly people. *Cochrane Database Syst Rev.* 2003:4;CD000340.

Herdman, S. *Vestibular Rehabilitation.* F.A. Davis Company: Philadelphia, PA;2000.

Haas EN ed; Handbook of Injury and Violence Prevention Atlanta GA, Springer 2007 Author of chapter. Chapter 3: Interventions to prevent falls among older adults. In: Haas, EN, ed. *Handbook of Injury and Violence Prevention*. Atlanta, GA:Springer;2007.

Nelson M, et al. Physical activity and public health in older adults: Recommendations from the American College of Sports Medicine and the American Heart Association. *Am J Sports Med*. 2007:39(8);1435-1445.

Nelson, ME. *Strong women stay young*. Bantam Books: New York, NY;2000.

Podsaidlo D, Richardson S. The timed up and go: A test of basic functional mobility for frail elderly persons. *Journal of the Am Geriatr Soc*. 1991:39;142-148.

Rikli RE, Jones CJ. *Senior fitness test manual human kinetics*: Champaign, IL;2001.

Rose, D. *Fall Proof: A comprehensive balance and mobility training program human kinetics*: Champaign, IL;2003.

Shumway-Cook A, Brauer S, Woollacott M. Predicting the probability of falls in community-dwelling older adults using the "Timed Up and Go Test." *Phys Ther*. 2000:80;896-903.

Tinetti ME. Performance-oriented assessment of mobility problems in elderly patients. *J Am Geriatr Soc*. 1986:34;119-126.

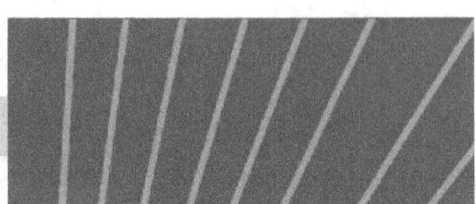

Building Block 3: Medication review and management

The purpose of medication review and management is to identify and eliminate medication side effects and interactions, such as dizziness or drowsiness, that can increase the risk of falls.

Many older adults are unaware that their daily medications may increase their fall risk. Aging affects the absorption, distribution, metabolism, and elimination of medications. Age can also increase sensitivity to potential side effects. Older adults may get prescriptions from multiple doctors. Fall risk increases with the total number of prescription and over-the-counter medications.

Psychoactive medications (drugs that alter brain function) increase fall risk. These include antidepressants, tranquilizers, antipsychotics, antianxiety drugs, and sleep medications. Other medications that may cause problems include those prescribed to treat seizure disorders, blood pressure-lowering medications, cholesterol-lowering medications, heart medications, and painkillers. A medication review checklist is included in Appendix F.

Drug side effects that can contribute to falling include blurred vision, hypotension leading to dizziness and lightheadedness, sedation, decreased alertness, confusion and impaired judgment, delirium, compromised neuromuscular function, and anxiety. Review and modification of the medication regimen by a healthcare provider can frequently reverse or minimize these effects.

Clinical practice recommendations include medication reviews by healthcare providers for older adults who have fallen.

Fall Intervention Studies that Include Medication Review and Management

PROFET (Prevention of Falls in the Elderly Trial) (Close, et al.)

Yale FICSIT (Frailty and Injuries: Cooperative Studies of Intervention Techniques) (Tinetti, et al.)

A Multifactorial Program (Wagner, et al.)

For more details, refer to the companion publication, Preventing Falls: What Works. A CDC Compendium of Effective Community-based Interventions from Around the World

PROGRAMS IN ACTION

California Department of Aging's Medication Management Program

The Medication Management Program is an evidence-based, federally funded program under Title IIID of the Older Americans Act. Funds are distributed to California Area Agencies on Aging to provide a wide variety of community-based services and information at multipurpose senior centers, at congregate meal sites, through home delivered meal programs and at other appropriate sites.

The purpose of the Medication Management Program is to improve the quality of life for older adults and prevent premature institutionalization by working with them to manage their use of over the counter and prescription medications, vitamin, mineral, and herbal supplements.

The target population for this program included individuals aged 60 years and over who live in an area of greatest economic need, who live in a medically underserved area of the region, or who have a chronic medical conditions that can improve with education and non-medical intervention.

The following are examples of the community-based activities and partnerships in this program:

- Pharmacists' or pharmacy students' presentations on how older adults can manage their medications, drug-nutrient interactions, and supplements. The presentation may include a personalized medication review to identify expired medications, answer client questions, and counsel older adults to assure they understand, are following directions, and taking medications properly. The pharmacists also encourage older adults to communicate with their doctors so they will be better informed about what medicines are being prescribed, why, and what results and/or side effects to expect.

- Partnerships with community-based organizations to provide "Rx Check Up" clinics.

- Distribution of passport size books for older adults to keep records of health and medications. Older adults can take the books with them to share with their doctors and pharmacist.

- Distribution of brochures related to medication management.

- Distribution of pill minders in various languages to help older adults manage their prescriptions.

- Information provided at Senior Health Fairs, through an Info Van, and through the Information and Assistance Program.

- Automated medication dispensers for frail and/or blind clients in their home.

For more information, visit www.aging.ca.gov/html/programs/medication_management.html

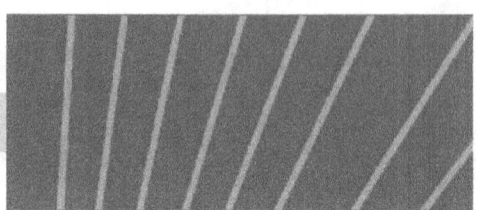

Tips for developing an effective medication review and management component

☐ Medication reviews are recommended for older people taking four or more medications and those taking any psychoactive medications.

☐ Medication reviews can be done in screening clinics, hospital programs, home visits by home health professionals, pharmacies, and doctors' offices.

☐ Medication reviews can be done by a pharmacist or a healthcare provider. Coordinated medication management that involves changing or reducing types or dosages of medications, should be done by the older adult's healthcare provider.

☐ Medication review and management may include assessing the need for vitamin D and calcium supplements as well as osteoporosis treatment.

☐ The amount and frequency of alcohol use should be included in a medication review.

Medication review and management web resources

National Institutes of Health Senior Health
nihseniorhealth.gov/takingmedicines/toc.html

American Geriatrics Society Clinical Guidelines for Prevention of Falls in Older Persons
www.americangeriatrics.org/products/positionpapers/Falls.pdf

Medications and falls in the elderly
www.pharmacists.ca/content/cpjpdfs/julaug04/July-August-FocusonPatientCareRevised.pdf

"10 questions to ask your doctor or pharmacist about your medications"
www.a4aa.com/Ten_Questions_to_Ask_Your_Doctor_or_Pharmacist_Outreach__2_.pdf

Building Block 4: Vision exams and vision improvement

Vision changes and vision loss associated with aging are common fall risk factors among older adults. Vision loss can contribute to falls by disturbing balance and by obscuring tripping and slipping hazards.

Many vision conditions, such as cataracts, glaucoma, and macular degeneration, are gradual and painless. However, if these conditions are diagnosed early, they can be managed to minimize vision loss.

Older adults may have difficulty learning about and/or accessing community programs that offer vision care services. CBOs can play an important role by providing information about and encouraging regular vision exams and care, and by referring older adults to community vision care services and resources.

Tips for developing an effective vision component

- ☐ Limited basic or simple vision screening can be performed by trained healthcare professionals such as physicians, nurse practitioners, physicians' assistants, registered nurses, and occupational therapists. However, basic vision screening does not identify all types of vision problems that need to be corrected.

- ☐ Comprehensive vision exams must be performed using specialized equipment. Therefore, these must be done by an optometrist or ophthalmologist.

- ☐ Medicare provides coverage for dilated eye exams, which are considered comprehensive vision exams.

Fall Prevention Intervention Studies that Include Vision Assessment

PROFET (Prevention of Falls in the Elderly Trial) (Close, et al.)
The NoFalls Intervention (Day, et al.)
A Multifactorial Program (Wagner, et al.)

For more details, refer to the companion publication, Preventing Falls: What Works. A CDC Compendium of Effective Community-based Interventions from Around the World

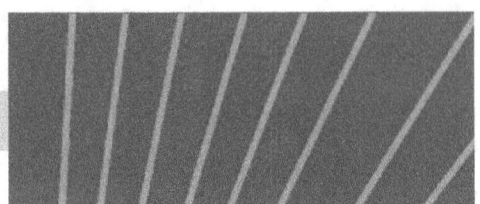

PROGRAMS IN ACTION

Vision Loss Resources

Vision Screening, Resource, and Education

Vision Loss Resources is an independent nonprofit 501 C(3) agency in Minneapolis, Minnesota. Its mission is to assist people who are blind or visually impaired achieve their full potential and to enrich the lives of all persons affected by blindness, vision loss, or hearing loss. Vision Loss Resources provides programs to enhance independent living and educate the community about vision loss.

Programs include:

- In-home assessment with service and resource plan development
- In-home vision evaluation for adaptive vision aids
- Hearing assessments with advocacy and resources for adaptive equipment
- Volunteers for assisting vision impaired clients to live independently
- Peer counseling and support and growth groups
- Leisure opportunities at the Vision Loss Resources' Community Center
- Life skills classes, training, and resources for maintaining independence
- Community and professional education about vision loss and resources
- Outreach and special projects providing resources and services for individuals and groups, with emphasis on special needs and cultural diversity.

For more information, Vision Loss Resources can be contacted by phone at 612.871.2222, on the web at www. visionlossresources.com, or e-mail at cleach@vlrw.org

Vision care is provided primarily by the following professionals:

☐ Optometrists examine people's eyes to diagnose vision problems and eye diseases, test patients' visual acuity, depth, and color perception, and test their ability to focus and coordinate their eyes. They prescribe eyeglasses and contact lenses and provide vision therapy and low vision rehabilitation.

☐ Ophthalmologists are physicians who perform detailed, comprehensive, and dilated vision exams and eye surgery. Like optometrists, they examine eyes and prescribe eyeglasses and contact lenses. They also diagnose and treat eye diseases and injuries.

- Dispensing opticians fit and adjust eyeglasses and, in some states, may fit contact lenses according to prescriptions written by ophthalmologists or optometrists.

- Local Area Agencies on Aging and state ophthalmology and optometry associations can provide information about community vision programs for older adults, for vision screening and/or exams, and financial assistance for vision needs.

- After the age of 60, vision assessments are recommended at least every 2 years, and more frequently if an eye condition has been diagnosed.

- Detailed eye exams by an optometrist or ophthalmologist are recommended at least once every 2 years for managing vision conditions and for corrective eye procedures, medications, and eyeglass prescriptions.

Vision web resources

National Institutes of Health Senior Health: Vision conditions and low vision topics
nihseniorhealth.gov/listoftopics.html

Medicare benefits for vision exams and vision care
www.medicare.gov

The American Academy of Ophthalmology
www.aao.org

The American Optometric Association
www.aoa.org

Opticians Association of America
www.oaa.org/index.shtml

National Eye Institute: Glaucoma—Resources for Patients and the Public
www.ski.org/Colenbrander/Images/Low_Vision_Exam.pdf
catalog.nei.nih.gov/productcart/pc/viewCat_L.asp?idCategory=78

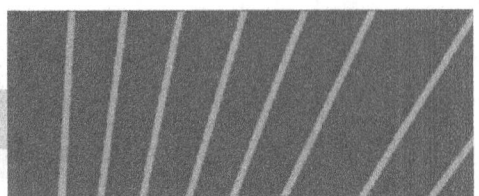

Building Block 5: Home safety assessment and home modification

Environmental factors play a part in approximately half of all falls that occur at home. Falls can be caused by slipping and tripping hazards, poor lighting, or the lack of needed home modifications such as bathroom grab bars, handicapped showers, stair railings, and ramps.

A home safety assessment can identify factors that may put an individual at risk for falling. Many older adults can benefit from home safety assessments, but those with a history of falls and/or with mobility or balance difficulties have the greatest need for such an assessment. Home assessments can be combined with or included with other direct one-on-one services that are provided by community service programs to residents in their homes.

Adult Fall Prevention Interventions with Home Safety Assessment & Modification Research Study Components

Home Visits by an Occupational Therapist (Cumming, et al.)
Falls-HIT (Home Intervention Team) Program (Nikolaus, et al.)
Stepping On (Clemson, et al.)
PROFET (Prevention of Falls in the Elderly Trial) (Close, et al.)
The NoFalls Intervention (Day, et al.)
The SAFE Health Behavior and Exercise Intervention (Hornbrook, et al.)
Yale FICSIT (Frailty and Injuries: Cooperative Studies of Intervention Techniques) (Tinetti, et al.)
A Multifactorial Program (Wagner, et al.)

For more details, refer to the companion publication, Preventing Falls: What Works. A CDC Compendium of Effective Community-based Interventions from Around the World

A self-administered home safety assessment checklist can be helpful if there is a plan for follow-up review with a trained professional to follow up and if information and referrals to home modification programs and resources are provided. *A Home Fall Prevention Checklist* is provided in Appendix G.

Older adults may have difficulty learning about and/or accessing home safety and home modification information and resources. Local Area Agencies on Aging (AAA) can provide information and referrals to local home modification programs. AAA can also provide information about state and federal programs that offer services and financial assistance to low-income seniors.

For an older adult who has been injured in a fall, Medicare may cover a home safety assessment and home modification if it is performed by an occupational or physical therapist. The senior must meet the home health reimbursement criteria, and these home services must be prescribed by a doctor, nurse practitioner, or physician assistant.

PROGRAMS IN ACTION

Pitt County Council on Aging: SPICE for Life

Senior Safety, Prevention, Intervention, and Community Education

This North Carolina fall prevention program's target population is low-income older adults, aged 60+, who are at high risk for loss of independence due to a decreased ability to function within the home. Fall risk factors typically addressed include:

- Home and environmental safety
- Medications
- Vision
- Mobility
- Lighting

Referrals for the program are called into the Pitt County Council on Aging (PCCOA) or are identified by PCCOA social workers. If the individual meets the criteria for the SPICE program and grant funding is available, a referral is sent to the program's lead occupational therapist (OT). The OT then further assesses eligibility and sets up an appointment for a home visit to perform a home modification and fall risk assessment.

SPICE makes use of two assessment tools that are standard to the program:

- A fall interview questionnaire to assess the individual
- A home safety modification assessment tool

Once the needs are identified, each low-income older adult who qualifies for the fall prevention/home safety program is educated about fall prevention strategies and provided with the necessary equipment and home modifications. When necessary, referrals for additional services are made to other service providers and agencies. Referral sources are varied (physicians, home health providers, aging network providers, etc.) and are continuing to increase as the community becomes more aware of the program. Community partnerships and involvement are critical elements of this program's success.

To contact the Pitt County Council on Aging, please call (252) 752-1717

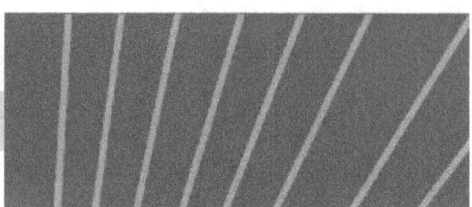

Occupational therapists can conduct environmental assessments, assess how the older adult interacts with their home environment, and suggest adaptations or modifications that can help older adults with limited physical function or low vision prevent falls and live independently.

Tips for developing an effective home safety component

☐ Home safety assessments and modifications are most effective when they are done in the home by an occupational therapist and when they include education, recommendations, and a follow-up home visit to assess the need for additional modifications.

☐ Home assessments and modifications by an occupational therapist are especially effective in reducing falls among older adults who have already had a fall.

☐ Occupational therapists are specifically trained to help individuals adapt their living environments to their physical needs, so they can perform their daily activities as independently and safely as possible. Occupational therapists are also trained to provide education to older adults, their family members, and caregivers.

☐ Trained professionals such as a Certified Aging in Place Specialist (certified by the National Association of Home Builders), registered nurses, and physical therapists can also effectively carry out home assessments and modifications, in collaboration with occupational therapists.

☐ In addition to home modifications, some older adults may need to use personal assistive safety and mobility devices. An occupational or physical therapist can provide the training needed to use these devices properly.

Home safety web resources

American Occupational Therapy Association's Fact Sheet on Occupational Therapy and Prevention of Falls

www.aota.org/Consumers/WhatisOT/FactSheets/
Conditions/39478.aspx

CDC's "Check for Safety: A Home Fall Prevention Checklist for Older Adults" brochure

www.cdc.gov/ncipc/duip/fallsmaterial.htm

National Resource Center on Supportive Housing and Home Modification

www.homemods.org

Home Safety Council: State of Home Safety's Facts About Safety in the Home

homesafetycouncil.org/state_of_home_safety/sohs_2004_p017.pdf

Home Safety Checklist (in English, Spanish, Chinese, Italian, Russian, Tagalog)

www.aging.ca.gov/resources/home_housing/home_safety_checklist.html

Ladder Safety Information Sheets

orthoinfo.aaos.org/fact/thr_report.cfm?Thread_
ID=92&topcategory=Injury%20Prevention

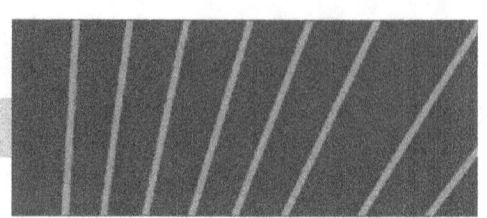

Notes:

Chapter 6

Evaluating Your
Fall Prevention Program

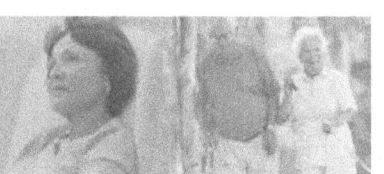

CDC's National Center for Injury Prevention and Control has developed recommended approaches for evaluating injury prevention programs, and these can be adapted for fall prevention programs. This chapter summarizes the key elements of these approaches. More complete and detailed information can be found in *Demonstrating Your Program's Worth: A Primer on Evaluation for Programs to Prevent Unintentional Injury* The full text of this publication can be found in either html format at **www.cdc.gov/ncipc/pub-res/demonstr.**

With objective evaluation, program managers can:

- Show that their program is benefiting
- Show funding agencies that their program is successful
- Produce facts and figures to demonstrate positive outcomes
- Share the results in publications and presentations to be more likely to receive continued funding

Evaluation should begin while the program is in the earliest development stages, not after the program is complete. Evaluation is an ongoing process that begins as soon as someone decides to develop and implement a program; it continues throughout the life of the program; and it ends with a final assessment of how well the program met or is meeting its goals. Goal setting is crucial to the evaluation of your program whether you measure the number of participants who complete an exercise program or the percent change in participants' knowledge about fall risk factors.

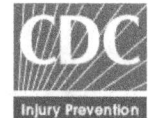

The earlier evaluation begins, the fewer mistakes are made and the greater the likelihood of success. In fact, for an injury prevention program to show success, evaluation must be an integral part of its design and operation and evaluation activities must be part of the program activities.

If a program is well designed and well run, evaluating the final results will be a straightforward task of analyzing information that is gathered while the program is in operation. The results will be extremely useful, not only to your own program, but to other community partners, similar organizations, and injury prevention programs.

The following sections will help clarify:

- Why evaluation is worth the resources and effort involved
- How to conduct an evaluation, and
- How to incorporate evaluation into fall prevention programs.

These guidelines will help program managers conduct basic evaluations. Refer to Appendix H for a complete program evaluation checklist.

Methods for conducting evaluation

There are two methods of program evaluation:

- Qualitative methods (information or opinions collected in narrative form, such as through open-ended questions or interviews)
- Quantitative methods (information collected objectively or in number form through tracking, counting, or measuring)

The basic information in this chapter provides enough information for you to conduct simple evaluations. However, some organizations may choose to hire an evaluation consultant. The *Demonstrating Your Program's Worth: A Primer on Evaluation for Programs to Prevent Unintentional Injury* publication also provides detailed information to enable you to communicate with, hire, and supervise evaluation consultants.

42

Summary of qualitative evaluation methods—personal interview

Method:

Personal interviews

Purpose:

1. To have individual, open-ended discussion on a range of issues.
2. To obtain in-depth information from individuals about their perceptions and concerns.

Number of People to Interview or Events to Observe:

The larger and more diverse the target population, the more people must be interviewed.

Resources Required:

- Trained interviewers
- Written guidelines for interviewer
- Recording equipment
- A transcriber
- A private location

Advantages:

- Can be used to discuss sensitive subjects that the interviewee may be reluctant to discuss in a group.
- Can probe individual experience in depth.
- Can be done by telephone.

Disadvantages:

- Time consuming to conduct interviews and analyze data.
- Transcription can be time-consuming and expensive.
- One-on-one interviews can lead participants to bias their answers toward "socially acceptable" responses.

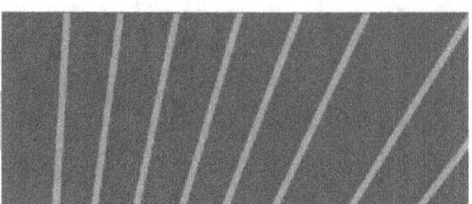

Summary of qualitative evaluation methods— focus group

Method:

Focus Groups

Purpose:

1. To have an open-ended group discussion on a range of issues.
2. To obtain in-depth information about perceptions and concerns from a group.

Number of People to Include:

4 to 8 participants per group.

Resources Required:

- Trained moderator(s)
- Appropriate meeting room
- Audio and/or visual recording equipment

Advantages:

- Can interview many people at once.
- Response from one group member can stimulate ideas of another.

Disadvantages:

- Individual responses can be influenced by group.
- Transcription can be expensive.
- Participants choose to attend and may not be representative of target population.
- Because of group pressure, participants may give "socially acceptable" responses.
- Focus groups are harder to coordinate than individual interviews.

Summary of qualitative evaluation methods— participant-observation

---

Method:

Participant-Observation

Purpose:

To see firsthand how an activity operates.

Number of Events to Observe:

The number of events to observe depends on the purpose. To evaluate people's behavior during a meeting may require observing only one event (meeting). However, to see if grab bars are installed correctly may require observing many events (installations).

Resources Required:

- Trained observers

Advantages:

- Provides firsthand knowledge of a situation.
- Can discover problems the people involved are unaware of (e.g., that their own actions in particular situations cause others to react negatively).
- Can determine whether products are being used properly (e.g., whether a walking device is being adjusted and used correctly).
- Can produce information from people who have difficulty verbalizing their points of view.

Disadvantages:

- Can affect the activity being observed.
- Can be time consuming.
- Can be labor intensive.

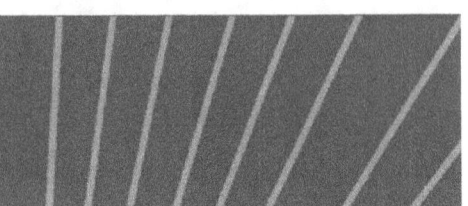

Summary of quantitative evaluation methods— counting system

Method:

Counting systems

Purpose:

1. To record the number of contacts with program participants (e.g., number of people attending each exercise class).
2. To record the number of contacts with people outside the program (e.g., number of meetings with partners).
3. To record the number of items a program distributes or receives (e.g., brochures and fact sheets).
4. To measure changes in people's knowledge, attitudes, beliefs, or behaviors by collecting the same information at the beginning and end of the program.
5. To estimate the amount spent on delivering your program.

The stages of evaluation

There are four stages of program evaluation:

- Formative
- Process
- Impact
- Outcome

The appropriate time to conduct each stage and the most suitable methods to use are outlined below.

Stage 1: Formative evaluation

- Whether proposed messages are likely to reach, to be understood by, and to be accepted by the people you are trying to serve (e.g., shows the strengths and weaknesses of proposed educational materials).
- How people in the target population get information (e.g., which newspapers they read or radio stations they listen to).
- Whom the target population respects as a spokesperson (e.g., a physician or local celebrity).
- Details that program developers may have overlooked about materials, strategies, or ways of distributing information (e.g., that seniors have difficulty reaching the location where classes are being held).

- During the development of a new program.
- When an existing program 1) is being modified, 2) has problems with no obvious solutions, or 3) is being used in a new setting, with a new population, or to target a new problem or behavior.

- Allows programs to make revisions before the full effort begins.
- Maximizes the likelihood that the program will succeed.

- Qualitative methods such as personal interviews with open-ended questions, focus groups, and participant observation.

(For details, see page 25 of *Demonstrating Your Program's Worth: A Primer on Evaluation for Programs to Prevent Unintentional Injury*)

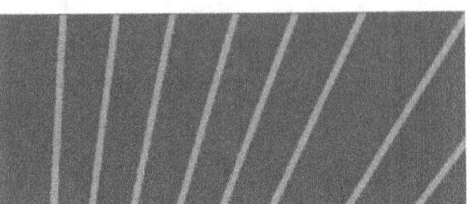

Stage 2: Process evaluation

- How well a program is working (e.g., how many people are participating in the program and how many people are not).
- Identifies early any problems that occur in reaching the target population.
- Allows programs to evaluate how well their plans, procedures, activities, and materials are working and to make adjustments before logistical or administrative weaknesses become entrenched.

When to use:

- As soon as the program begins operation.

Why it is useful:

- Allows programs to make revisions before the full effort begins.
- Maximizes the likelihood that the program will succeed.

Methods to use:

- Quantitative methods, such as:
  - Tracking direct contacts with all who are served by the program (older adults who have had direct contact with the program, the nature of the direct contacts, number of educational brochures distributed).
  - Tracking indirect contacts (through health care providers, adult children of older adults, or other organizations who are sharing information with older adults).

(For details, see page 27 of *Demonstrating Your Program's Worth: A Primer on Evaluation for Programs to Prevent Unintentional Injury*)

Stage 3: Impact evaluation

- The degree to which a program is meeting its intermediate goals (e.g., how awareness about the value of exercise or home safety has changed among program participants).
- Changes in the target population's knowledge, attitudes, beliefs, or measurable fall risk factors.

When to use:

- When the program is being implemented and has made contact with at least one person or one group of people in the target population.

Why it is useful:

- Allows management to modify materials or move resources from a nonproductive to a productive area of the program.
- Tells programs whether they are moving toward achieving their goals.

Methods to use:

- Baseline measurement: measuring the target population's knowledge, attitudes, beliefs, behaviors, or health risk factor (such as muscle strength or balance) before beginning the program or receiving services, using surveys and/or objective participant assessments.
- Progress measurement: measuring the target population's knowledge, attitudes, beliefs, behaviors or health risk factors (such as muscle strength or balance) at a predetermined amount of time such as at the end of a 3-month exercise class or at regular intervals in an ongoing program. Measurements can be made using surveys and/or objective participant assessments.

(For details, see page 29 of *Demonstrating Your Program's Worth: A Primer on Evaluation for Programs to Prevent Unintentional Injury*)

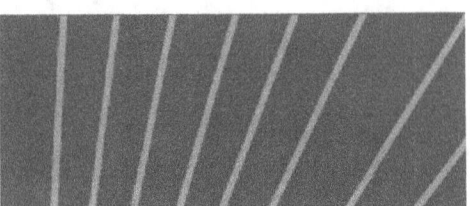

Stage 4: Outcome evaluation

- The degree to which the program has met its ultimate goals (e.g., how much an exercise and education program has improved a person's ability to carry out daily activities and reduce fall risks).

When to use:

- For ongoing programs (e.g., group exercise classes offered throughout the year) at appropriate intervals.
- For one-time programs (e.g., a 6-month program to conduct home safety assessments and distribute home modification equipment or devices) when program is complete.

Why it is useful:

- Allows programs to learn from their successes and failures and to incorporate what they have learned into the program or into their next project.
- Provides evidence of success for use in future budget development and requests for funding.

Methods to use:

- Generally the same methods used in impact evaluation are used in outcome evaluation.

(For details, see page 32 of *Demonstrating Your Program's Worth: A Primer on Evaluation for Programs to Prevent Unintentional Injury*)

Determining which stage to use

To find out which stage of evaluation your program is ready for, answer the questions below. Then follow the directions provided after the answer.

Q. *Does your program meet any of the following criteria?*

- It is just being planned and you want to determine how best to operate.
- It has some problems you do not know how to solve.
- It has just been modified and you want to know whether the modifications work.
- It has just been adapted for a new setting, population, problem, or behavior.

If yes to any of the four criteria, begin formative evaluation.

If no to all criteria, read the next question.

Q. *Your program is now in operation. Do you have information on who is being served, who is not being served, and how much service you are providing?*

If yes, read the next question.

If no, begin process evaluation. You may also be ready for impact evaluation. Read the next question.

Q. *Your program has completed at least one encounter with one member or one group in the target population (e.g., completed one exercise class). Have you measured the results of that encounter?*

If yes, read the next question.

If no, you are ready for impact evaluation. If you believe you have had enough encounters to allow you to measure your success in meeting your overall program goals, read the next question.

Q. *Is your program complete?*

If yes, you are ready for outcome evaluation.

If no, reread the above questions or refer to the publication in *Demonstrating Your Program's Worth: A Primer on Evaluation for Programs to Prevent Unintentional Injury.* If you are still uncertain, consult a professional.

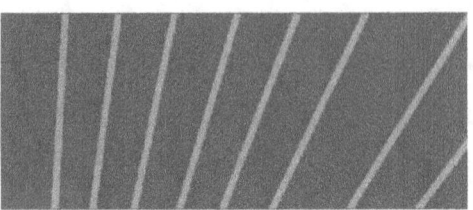

Evaluation web resources

Thompson NJ, McClintock HO. Demonstrating Your Program's Worth: A Primer on Evaluation for Programs To Prevent Unintentional Injury. Atlanta: Centers for Disease Control and Prevention, National Center for Injury Prevention and Control, 1998; revised March 2000.
www.cdc.gov/ncipc/pub-res/demonstr.htm

British Columbia Research Institute for Children's & Women's Health, Injury Prevention Program Evaluation Manual
www.injuryresearch.bc.ca/Publications/Reports/ProgEvalMan%20 Report.pdf

National Council on Aging's Evidence-based Healthy Aging Programming: Tools and Checklists
healthyagingprograms.org/content.asp?sectionid=32&ElementID=439

CDC Evaluation Working Group: resources for project evaluation
www.cdc.gov/eval/resources.htm

RE-AIM Evaluation Framework
www.re-aim.org/2003/commleader.html

Basic Guide to Outcomes Based Evaluation for Nonprofit Organizations with Very Limited Resources
www.managementhelp.org/evaluatn/outcomes.htm

Chapter 7

Promoting Your Fall Prevention Program

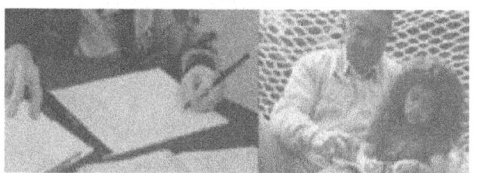

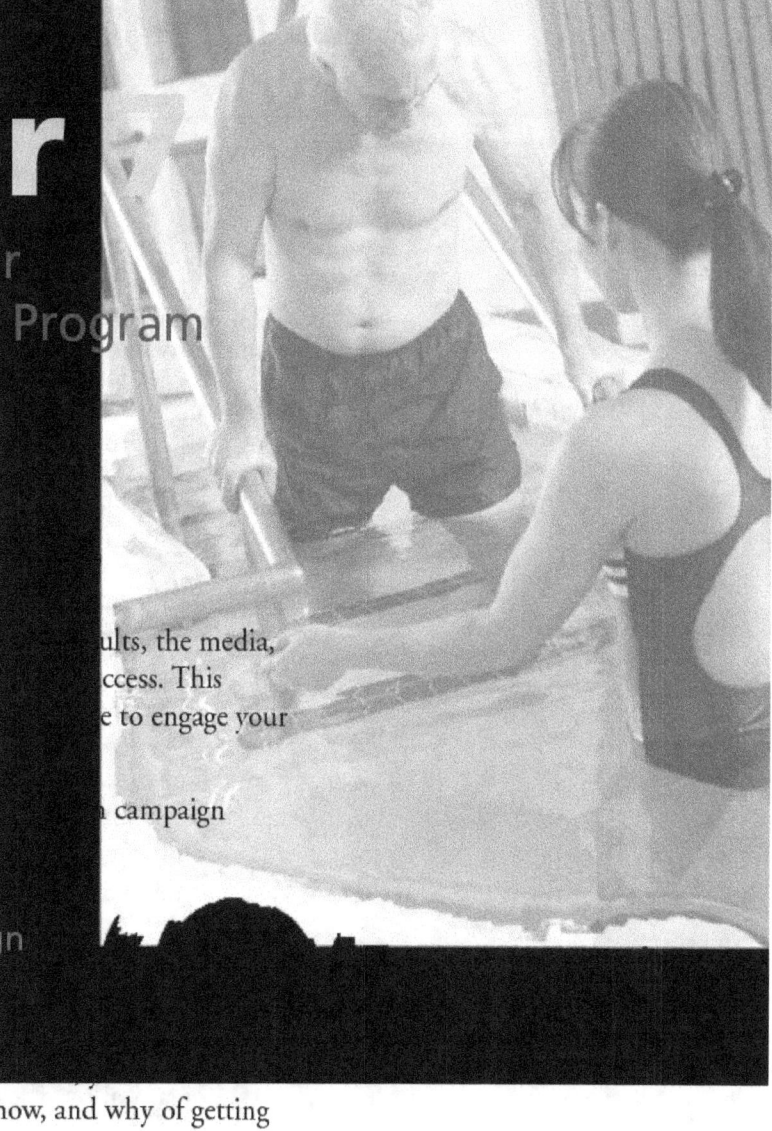

Publicizing your fall prevention program to [older ad]ults, the media, and others in the community will be critica[l to its su]ccess. This chapter provides tips and techniques that y[ou can us]e to engage your community in fall prevention by:

- Conducting a successful community [outreac]h campaign
- Working with the media

Conducting a successful campaign

The word "campaign" applies to a public he[alth effort of] any size. Even if you are only developing a [flyer about a] new home-based exercise program for olde[r adults, you need] to determine the who, what, when, where, how, and why of getting the flyer written, designed, printed, and distributed so that it will effectively reach your target audience.

This section provides an overview of campaign development, from concept through evaluation. For more detailed information on the theory and application of health communication, visit the CDC National Center for Health Marketing website shown at the end of this section.

The eight steps outlined below will help you make the best use of your limited time and resources in developing a successful community outreach campaign.

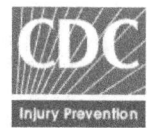

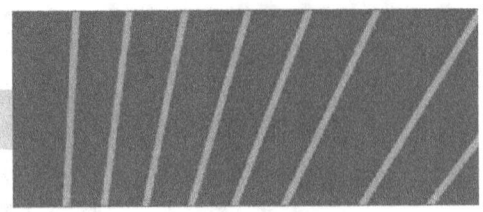

Step 1: Assess your current situation. Take a realistic look at your community and ask pertinent questions.

☐ Is your community concerned about fall prevention or will you need to lay some educational groundwork?

☐ Do you believe your local media (radio, TV, newspaper, websites) would support your campaign?

☐ What resources do you have that can help your efforts?

☐ Would a campaign be easier to mount if you partnered with other organizations in your community who serve older adults?

Step 2: Set your campaign goal and objectives. Identify the goals and objectives for your outreach campaign. A goal is the overall health improvement you hope to achieve, such as reducing falls among older adults in your community. An objective is a specific outcome that you can use to measure progress toward your goal.

Set realistic and measurable objectives. For example:

☐ Double the enrollment of your exercise classes for seniors.

☐ Increase the percentage of older adults served by your organization who have installed grab bars or railings.

Step 3: Identify the target audiences your campaign should reach. Identify the groups of people you need to reach to meet the goal you set in Step 2. Learn as much as you can about them. Remember that the needs, beliefs, values, and expectations of target audiences vary.

☐ Do the older adults you wish to reach see themselves as active and youthful?

☐ Are they committed to living independently?

☐ Should you reach out to adult children of older adults or healthcare providers in your campaign?

The more you know about your target audience, the more effectively you can tailor your promotional efforts. For example, the Internet may not be an effective way to reach certain groups of older adults.

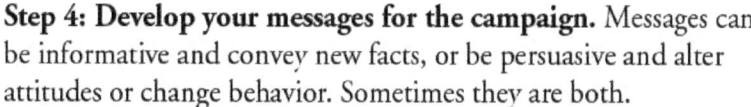

Step 4: Develop your messages for the campaign. Messages can be informative and convey new facts, or be persuasive and alter attitudes or change behavior. Sometimes they are both.

☐ Many messages begin by raising awareness about an issue or program so people can agree with it, understand it, believe it, and then eventually act on it.

☐ Consider gender, culture, and age groups. Messages aimed at people aged 60 to 70 should be framed differently from those for individuals over 70. If the older adults you want to reach perceive themselves as youthful, they may ignore a message about the health problems of aging. A message focused on "staying healthy and independent" may generate more positive response than one focused on "preventing hip fractures and other injuries."

☐ Pretest your messages with a sample of the audience and see if your message appeals to them.

☐ Use audience feedback to make adjustments before launching your campaign.

Step 5: Identify message outlets. Decide how you can deliver your message most effectively. Answers to the following questions can help you identify the best outlets for your message.

☐ Where does your audience get information that they trust? Is it from the media, their peers, their physicians, or children?

☐ Where does your audience spend time? Do they spend time at senior centers, libraries, or faith-based organizations such as churchs or synagogues?

Partnerships offer unique opportunities to reach complementary target audiences. Healthcare providers can publicize your fall prevention program to older adults. Providers also can directly refer high-risk adults to your program. When asking a partner to help with promotional activities, emphasize the connection between their work and your program goal. See Appendix I for a sample letter to healthcare providers to solicit referrals.

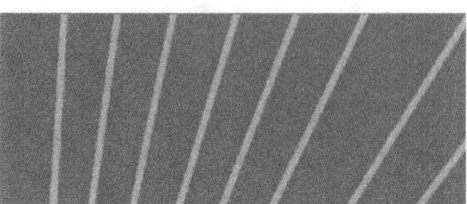

Step 6: Develop an action plan for the campaign. Create an action plan that demonstrates good time and resource management. While it can be simple or complex, at a minimum your action plan should identify:

- ☐ Major activities and tasks

- ☐ Target date for completing each task

- ☐ The person responsible for ensuring that each task is completed

Step 7: Develop and pretest campaign materials. In developing materials, pay attention to reading level, print size, and languages.

- ☐ Keep your wording simple and direct.

- ☐ Consider design as well as content. For example, older adults may prefer larger type.

- ☐ Pretest any materials you develop as part of your campaign with members of your target audience group and make modifications based on their feedback.

This crucial step can make the difference between success and failure in a community outreach campaign.

Step 8: Implement, evaluate, and modify your campaign. As you carry on your outreach campaign, determine if you are moving toward your goal. If not, investigate the reasons why.

- ☐ See what barriers are preventing the message from reaching the target audience.

- ☐ Determine what you can do to remove these obstacles.

- ☐ Use what you learn to improve your campaign.

Working with the media

You can use media such as local newspapers, radio, and television stations, to enhance your promotion activities. The media has a mandate to be of public service, so they should welcome the opportunity to make the community aware of your organization's fall prevention program. See your relationship with the media as one of mutual advantage; you provide useful and timely information for their audiences, and they provide public access and outreach for you.

☐ Start with your local telephone directory and create a list of media names and contact information for local reporters, especially the health reporter.

☐ Check with your library or bookstore to find media directories that list daily and weekly newspapers, television stations, radio stations, newswire services, Internet news outlets, magazines, newsletters, and business trade publications in your community. Some examples of media directories include Bacon's MediaSource and the News Media Yellow Book. (These web links can be found at the end of this section.)

☐ Don't overlook community newspapers as potential news outlets.

☐ Local organizations such as faith-based, and senior citizen groups that publish their own newsletters may be eager to publicize your prevention program.

☐ Develop key points to include in the media materials. Highlight the importance of your fall prevention program. If you're hosting a community event, offer key points to guest speakers in advance so they can include them in their remarks. Appendix J has key points that include facts and national statistics about falls among older adults. For a greater effect, try to include statistics about falls among older adults in your state or community. These statistics may be available from state and county health departments and local hospitals.

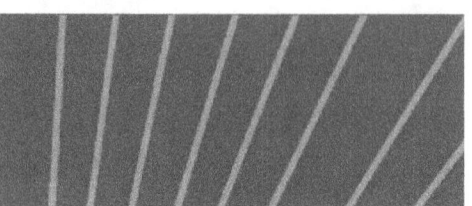

Promotional web resources

CDC National Center for Health Marketing
www.cdc.gov/healthmarketing

CISION
us.cision.com

News Media Yellow Book
www.leadershipdirectories.com/products/nmyb.htm

Chapter 8

Sustaining Your
Fall Prevention Program

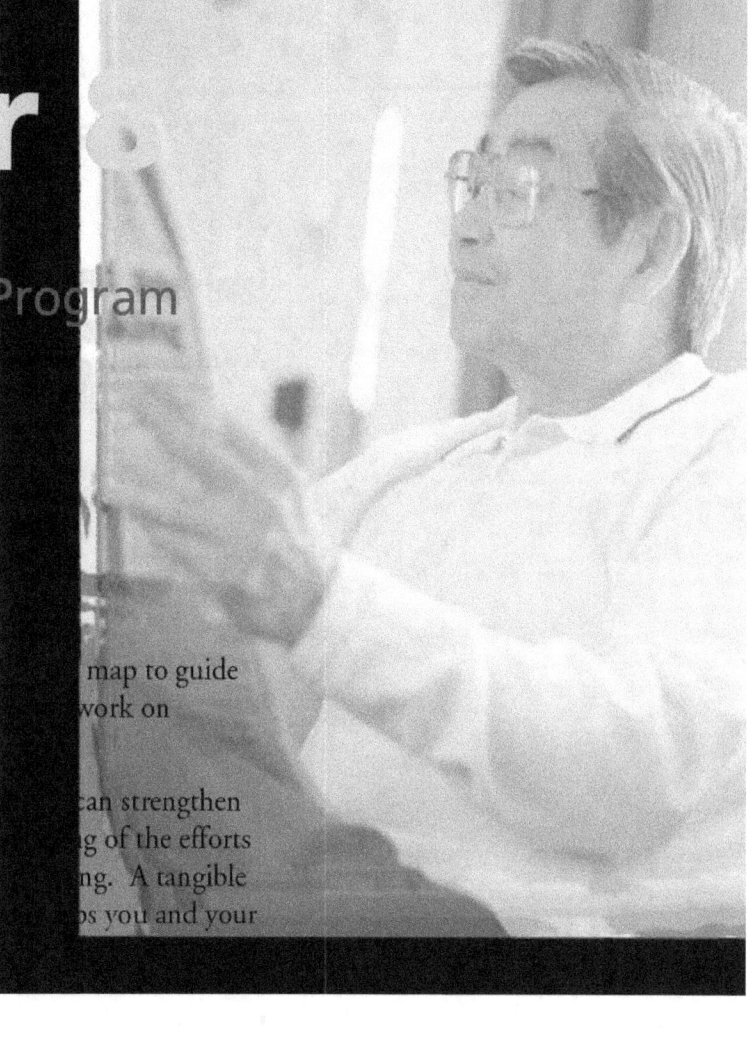

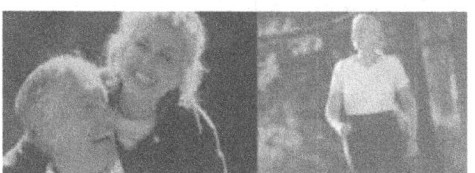

Create a written sustainability plan to provide a map to guide you and your program's community partners as you work on sustainability efforts.

The process of creating a written sustainability plan can strengthen community partners' commitment and understanding of the efforts needed to keep your program operating and improving. A tangible document that describes your sustainability plan helps you and your community partners monitor progress on sustainability. When developing your plan, consider the following:

Establish your vision

Determine the vision of your program. A common vision unifies all of your program's sustainability efforts. Write it down and share it with all involved. Keeping your vision in sight will serve to strengthen your program's sustainability.

Build collaboration

Continue to look for new community partners who possess unique skills and resources that will contribute to your program. Expanding your base of support is crucial to sustaining your program and providing its benefits to the older adults in your community.

Advocate for support

Seek advocates for your program among business leaders, other CBOs, and government representatives who will speak up and take action on behalf of your program.

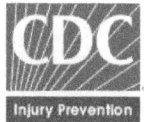

Integrate your program into community healthcare and senior services by linking with senior service providers, the health department, healthcare organizations, and the local Area Agency on Aging; they can provide ongoing community support and referrals.

Find funding

Secure diversified funding streams from public and private sources to increase your program's sustainability. Sources of funding include:

- Medicare
- Health Maintenance Organizations
- Private or managed care insurers
- Private organizations
- Federal/state/local government or agency
- Local, state, or national (public or private) grant funders
- Program participant fees

Use your program evaluation results to promote sustainability. Study your program goals and evaluation results to identify areas for improvement or change that might make your program more sustainable.

Demonstrate the benefits of your program. Share your evaluation results with your target audience, the community, your partners, your current and potential funding sources, and stakeholders.

See Attachment K for a template to help you create a sustainability plan for your fall prevention program.

Appendix A

Sample Individual
Falls Risk Assessment

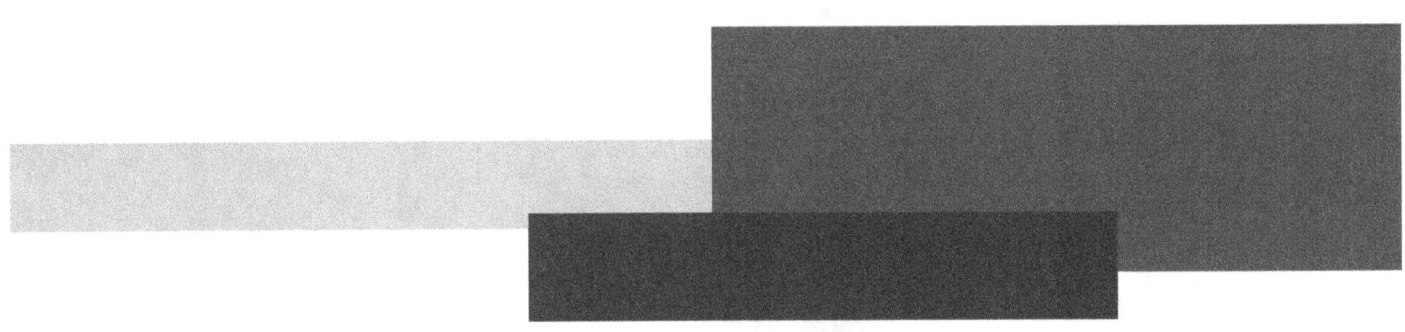

My Falls-Free Plan

Name: _____ Date: _____

As we grow older, gradual health changes and some medications can cause falls, but many falls can be prevented. Use this to learn what to do to stay active, independent, and falls-free.

Check "Yes" if you experience this (even if only **sometimes**)	No	Yes	What to do if you checked "Yes"
Have you had **any falls in the last six months**?			☐ Talk with your doctor(s) about your falls and/or concerns. ☐ Show this checklist to your doctor(s) to help understand and treat your risks, and protect yourself from falls.
Do you take **four or more** prescription or over-the-counter medications daily?			☐ Review your medications with your doctor(s) **and** your pharmacist at each visit, and with each new prescription. ☐ Ask which of your medications can cause drowsiness, dizziness, or weakness as a side effect. ☐ Talk with your doctor about anything that could be a medication side effect or interaction.
Do you have **any difficulty walking or standing**?			☐ Tell your doctor(s) if you have any pain, aching, soreness, stiffness, weakness, swelling, or numbness in your legs or feet—**don't ignore** these types of health problems. ☐ Tell your doctor(s) about **any** difficulty walking to discuss treatment. ☐ Ask your doctor(s) if physical therapy or treatment by a medical specialist would be helpful to your problem.
Do you use a **cane, walker, or crutches**, or have to hold onto things when you walk?			☐ Ask your doctor for training from a physical therapist to learn what type of device is best for you, and how to safely use it.
Do you have to **use your arms to be able to stand up from a chair**?			☐ Ask your doctor for a physical therapy referral to learn exercises to strengthen your leg muscles. ☐ Exercise at least two or three times a week for 30 min.
Do you ever feel **unsteady on your feet, weak, or dizzy**?			☐ Tell your doctor, and ask if treatment by a specialist or physical therapist would help improve your condition. ☐ Review all of your medications with your doctor(s) or pharmacist if you notice **any** of these conditions.
Has it been **more than two years since you had an eye exam**?			☐ Schedule an eye exam every two years to protect your eyesight and your balance.
Has your **hearing gotten worse with age**, or do your family or friends say you have a hearing problem?			☐ Schedule a hearing test every two years. ☐ If hearing aids are recommended, learn **how** to use them to help protect and restore your hearing, which helps improve and protect your balance.
Do you usually **exercise less than two days a week**? (for 30 minutes total each of the days you exercise)			☐ Ask your doctor(s) what types of exercise would be good for improving your strength and balance. ☐ Find some activities that you enjoy and people to exercise with two or three days/week for 30 min.
Do you drink **any alcohol** daily?			☐ Limit your alcohol to one drink per day to avoid falls.
Do you have **more than three chronic health conditions**? (such as heart or lung problems, diabetes, high blood pressure, arthritis, etc. Ask your doctor(s) if you are unsure.)			☐ See your doctor(s) as often as recommended to keep your health in good condition. ☐ Ask your doctor(s) what you should do to stay healthy and active with your health conditions. ☐ Report any health changes that cause weakness or illness as soon as possible.

The more "Yes" answers you have, the greater your chance of having a fall. **Be aware of what can cause falls, and take care of yourself to stay independent and falls-free!**

Reviewed by: _____

Appendix B

Identifying Partners Worksheet

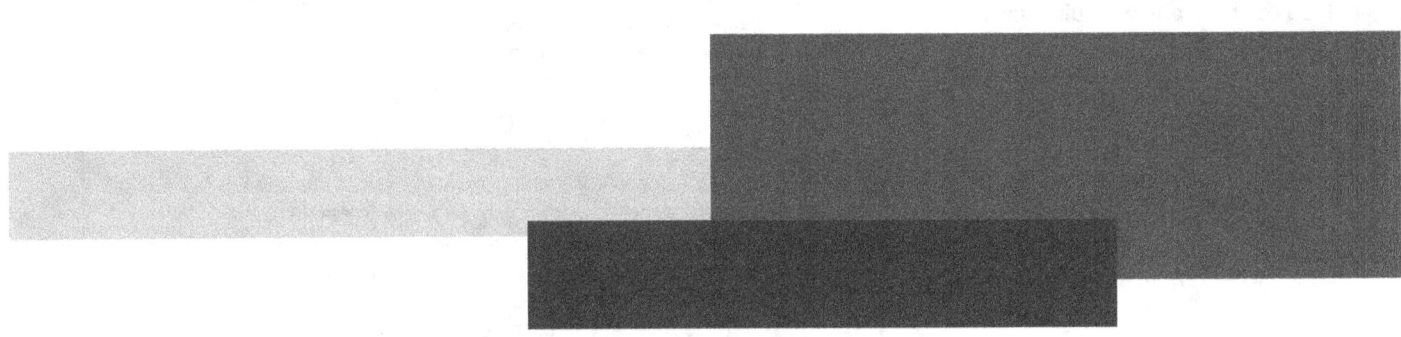

Appendix B - Identifying Potential Partners

Community Partners/ Resources	Fall Prevention Intervention Components						
	Education • Group • Individual	Assessment • Gait • Balance; simple • Balance; in-depth • Strength	Exercise • 1:1 balance alone • 1:1 strength with balance training • Group class • Individualized exercise/PT • Tai Chi	Medication • Medication review • Medication management	Vision • Basic assessment • Detailed assessment • Vision correction	Home Safety • Assessment • Basic modification** • Skilled modification**	Other • Assistive device training
Area Agency on Aging							
Community health care providers							
Community hospital (s) outpatient programs and services							
EMS/Trauma Injury Prevention Coordinator							
Fire Depts.							
Gym/fitness center							
Health Department							
Home health agency							
Home modification resources							
Library system							
Local service organization(s)							
Other resources							
Parks and recreation							
Pharmacy							
Physical/occupational therapy clinics							
University/ Community College							
YMCA							

Appendix C

Sample Fall Prevention Brochure

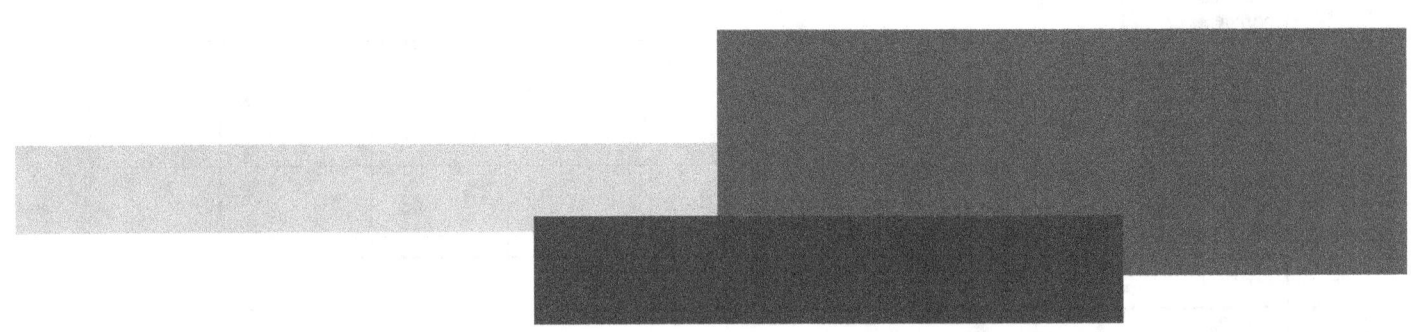

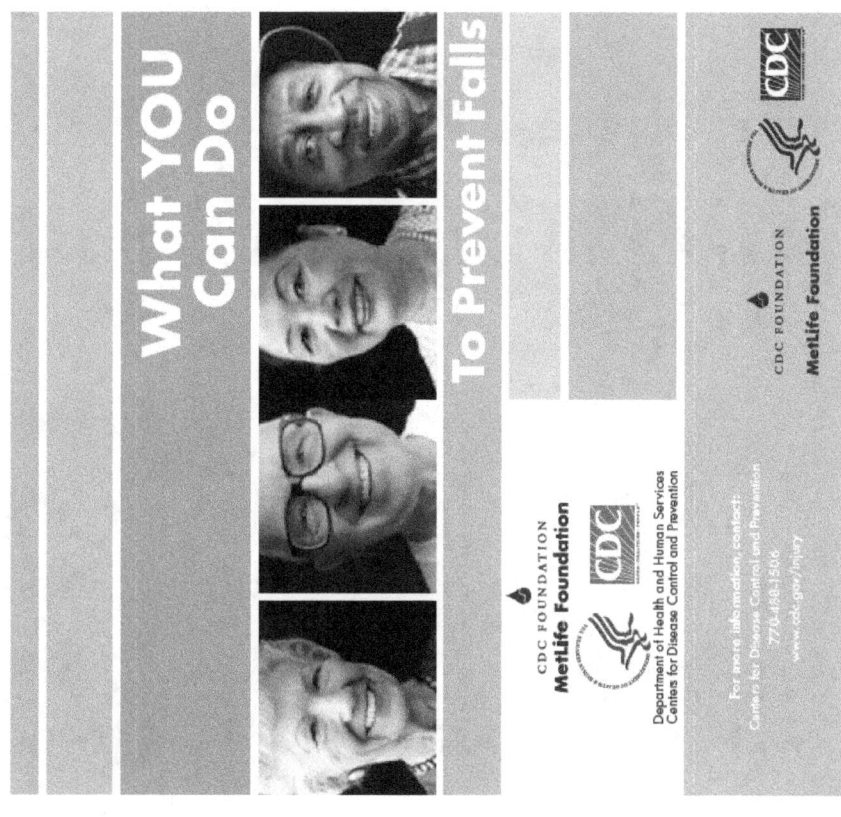

What YOU Can Do

To Prevent Falls

CDC FOUNDATION
MetLife Foundation

Department of Health and Human Services
Centers for Disease Control and Prevention

For more information, contact:
Centers for Disease Control and Prevention
770-488-1506
www.cdc.gov/injury

CDC FOUNDATION
MetLife Foundation

Many falls can be prevented. By making some changes, you can lower your chances of falling.

Four things YOU can do to prevent falls:

1. **Begin a regular exercise program**

2. **Have your health care provider review your medicines**

3. **Have your vision checked**

4. **Make your home safer**

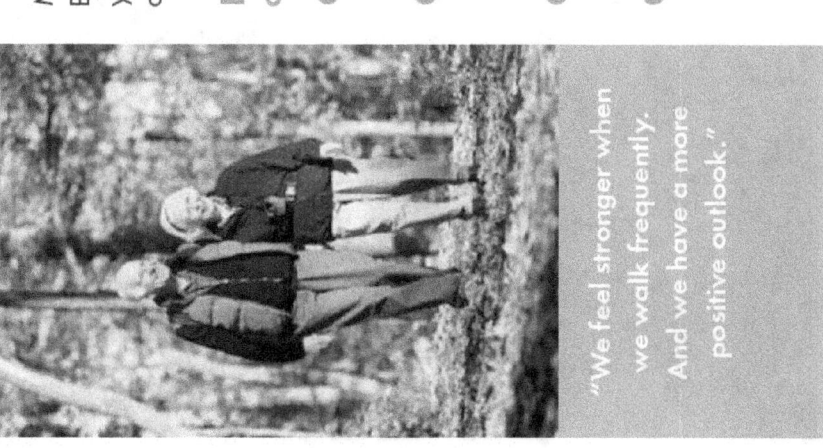

"We feel stronger when we walk frequently. And we have a more positive outlook."

Four things YOU can do to prevent falls:

❶ Begin a regular exercise program

Exercise is one of the most important ways to lower your chances of falling. It makes you stronger and helps you feel better. Exercises that improve balance and coordination (like Tai Chi) are the most helpful.

Lack of exercise leads to weakness and increases your chances of falling.

Ask your doctor or health care provider about the best type of exercise program for you.

"I thought I was too old to learn Tai Chi. But I enjoy the classes and my balance is much better."

❷ Have your health care provider review your medicines

Have your doctor or pharmacist review all the medicines you take, even over-the-counter medicines. As you get older, the way medicines work in your body can change. Some medicines, or combinations of medicines, can make you sleepy or dizzy and can cause you to fall.

❸ Have your vision checked

Have your eyes checked by an eye doctor at least once a year. You may be wearing the wrong glasses or have a condition like glaucoma or cataracts that limits your vision. Poor vision can increase your chances of falling.

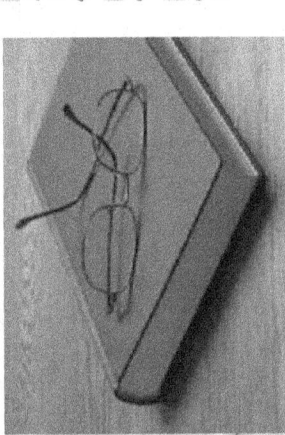
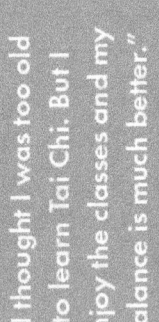
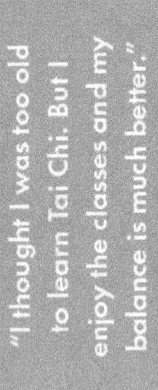

❹ Make your home safer

About half of all falls happen at home. To make your home safer:

☐ Remove things you can trip over (like papers, books, clothes, and shoes) from stairs and places where you walk.

☐ Remove small throw rugs or use double-sided tape to keep the rugs from slipping.

☐ Keep items you use often in cabinets you can reach easily without using a step stool.

☐ Have grab bars put in next to your toilet and in the tub or shower.

☐ Use non-slip mats in the bathtub and on shower floors.

☐ Improve the lighting in your home. As you get older, you need brighter lights to see well. Hang light-weight curtains or shades to reduce glare.

☐ Have handrails and lights put in on all staircases.

☐ Wear shoes both inside and outside the house. Avoid going barefoot or wearing slippers.

Appendix D

Sample Fall Prevention Presentation

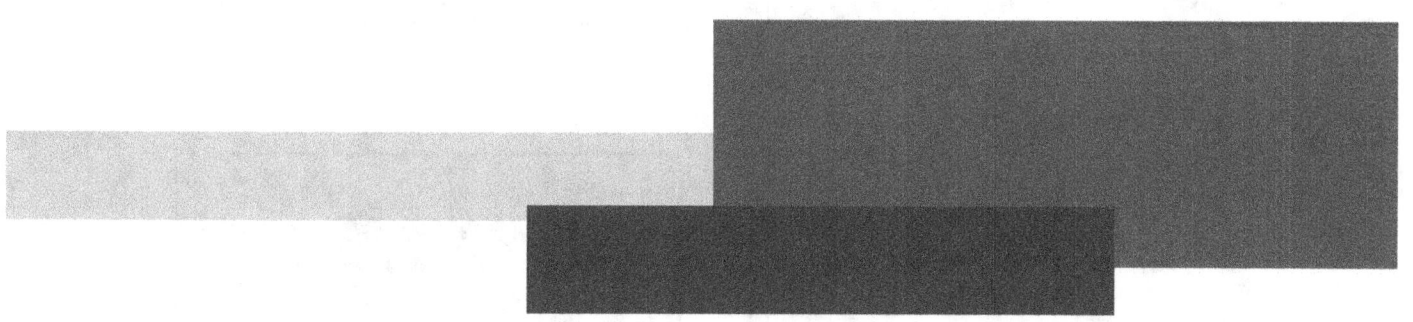

Appendix D - Fall Prevention PPT Thumbnails

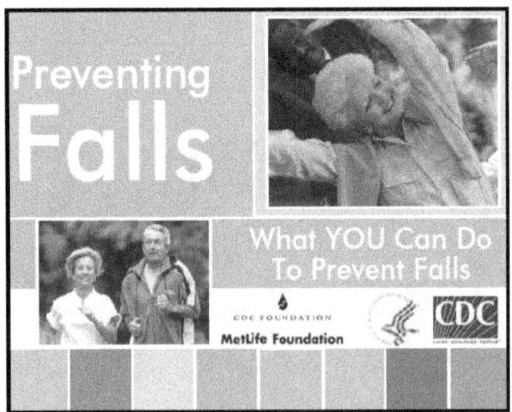

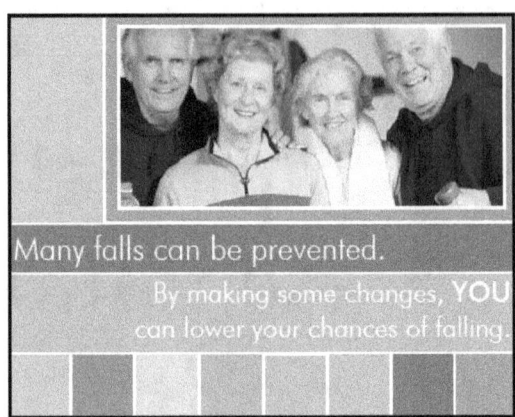

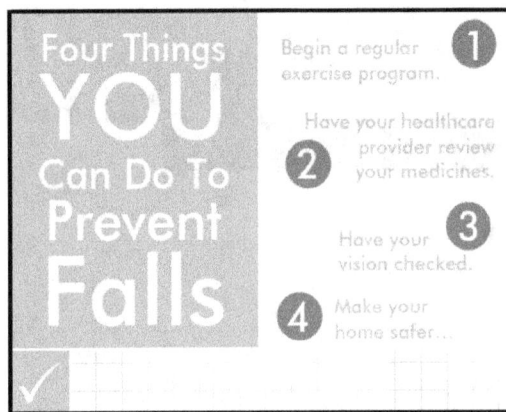

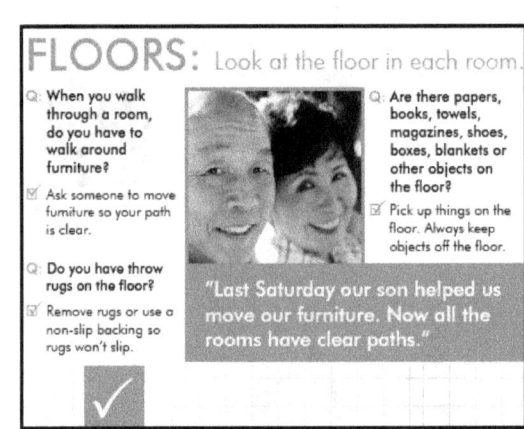

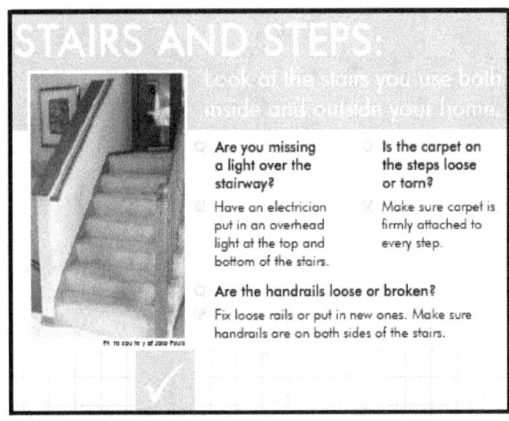

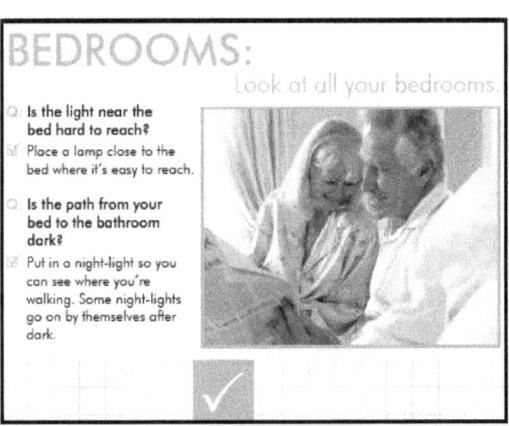

Appendix D - Fall Prevention PPT Thumbnails

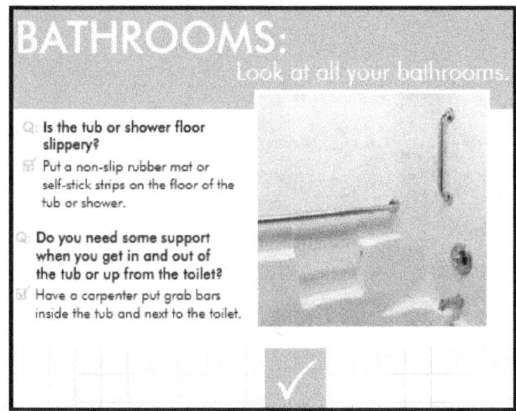

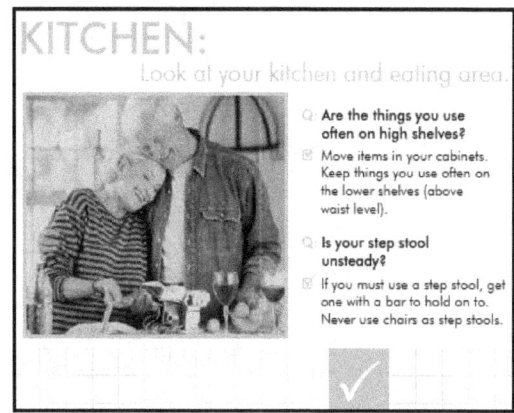

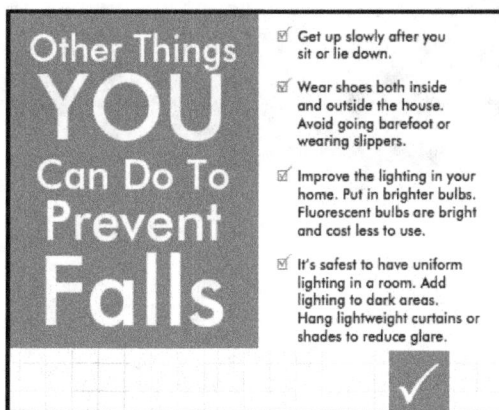

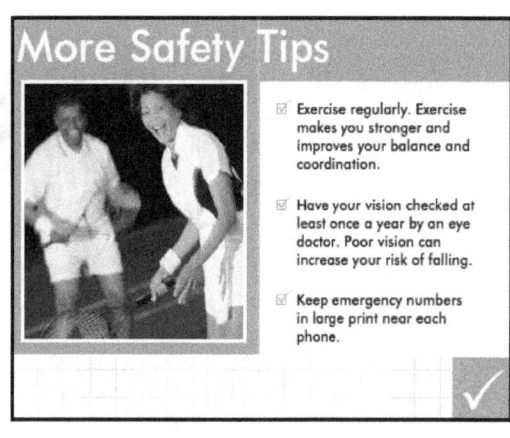

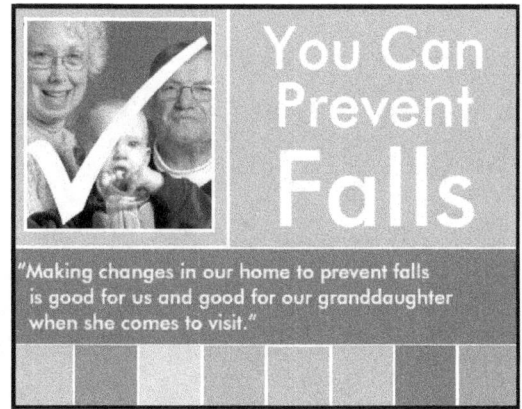

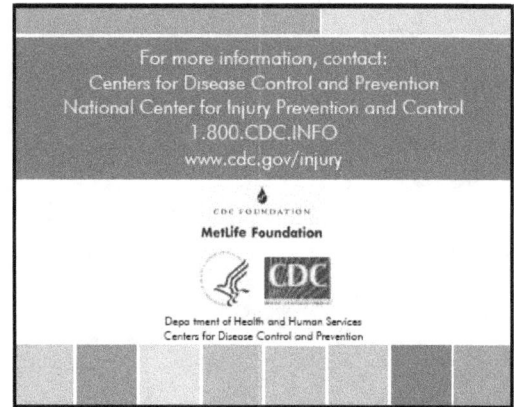

Appendix E
Sample Exercises

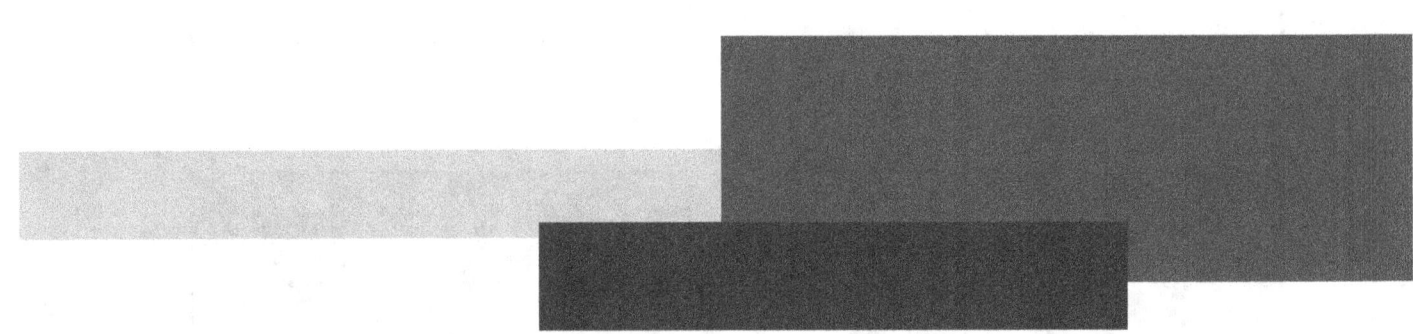

Stay Safe Stay Active
Daily Exercise Program

1. Warm up
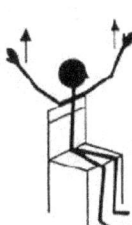

2. Shoulder rolls (Flexibility)
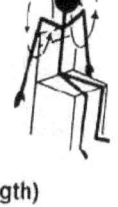

3. March on spot (mobility)
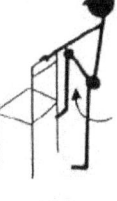

4. Ankle (strength)

5. Knee bend (strength)

6. Sit to Stand (strength)
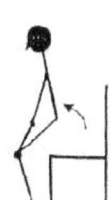

7. Calf (stretch)
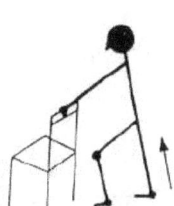

8. Calf (stretch)
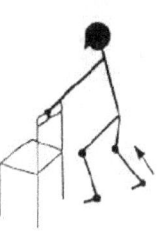

Thank you Sally Castell for your diagrams

Stay Safe Stay Active
Daily Exercise Program (Stage 2)

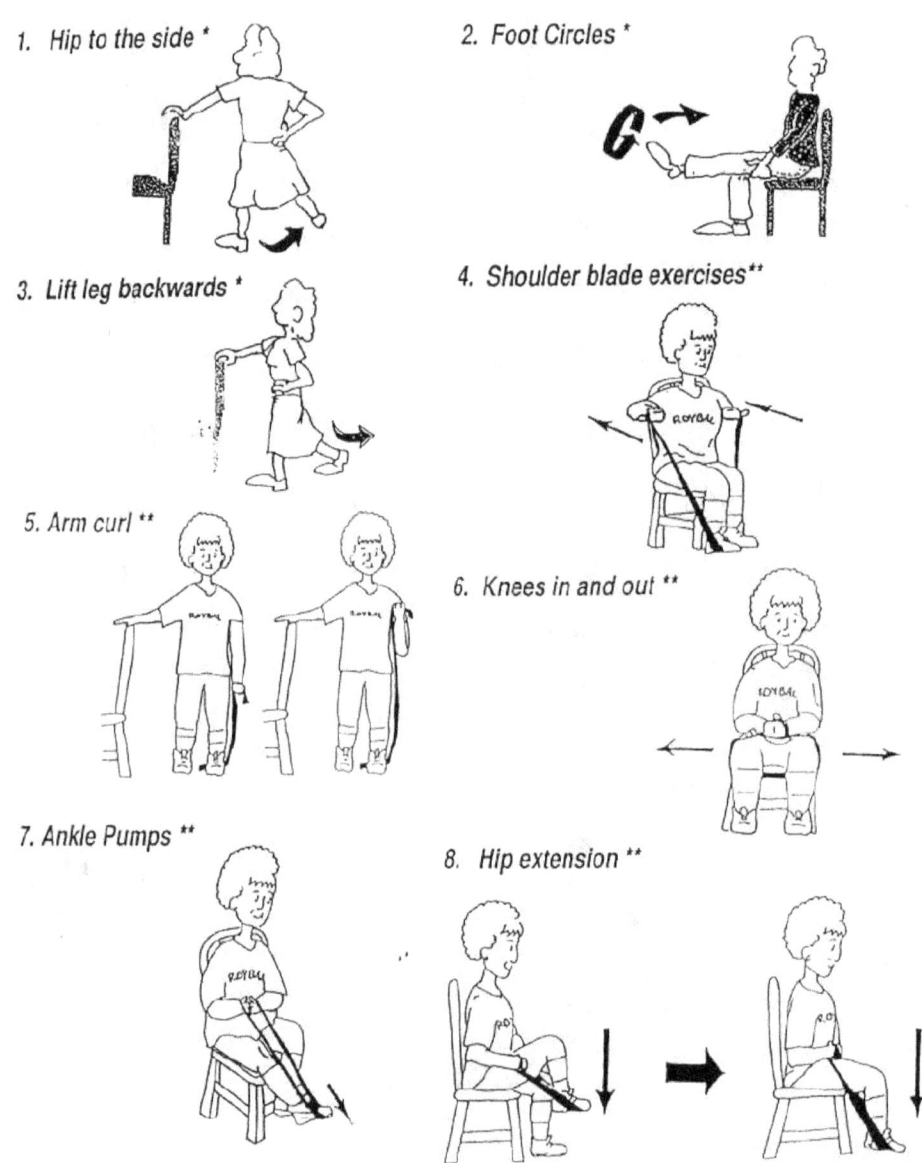

1. Hip to the side *

2. Foot Circles *

3. Lift leg backwards *

4. Shoulder blade exercises **

5. Arm curl **

6. Knees in and out **

7. Ankle Pumps **

8. Hip extension **

Thank you to Stay on Your Feet* and Roybal - Boston University** for allowing us to use your diagrams

Appendix F

Sample Medication Review Form

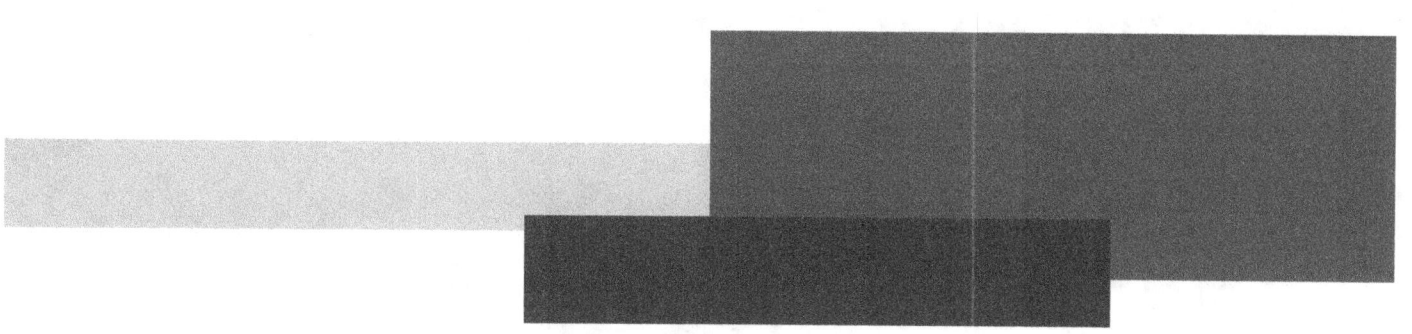

Appendix F - Fall Prevention Medication Review Checklist

Patient Name: _____ Review Date: _____

Number of medications patient was taking: _____

Please indicate which of the following recommendations were made/actions taken when reviewing the above patient's medication intake.

☐ Decrease number of medications, if possible (especially if taking more than four medications).
Notes:

☐ Investigate lower dosages of medications, especially psychotropic drugs, diuretics and cardiovascular drugs.
 Notes:

☐ Consider withdrawal of digoxin:
- In patients with stable CHF
- If CHF is due to valvular disease or hypertension
- If there is no response to digoxin after one month with decreased heart size, or increased exercise capacity
Notes:

☐ Stop or decrease number of psychotropic medications
- Neuroleptics (i.e., Phenothiazines, Butyrophenones)
- Sedative/hypnotics (i.e., Barbiturates, Hydroxyzine)
  - Antidepressants (i.e., Tricyclic Antidepressants, Selective Serotonin Uptake Inhibitors (SSRIs)
  - Benzodiazepines
Notes:

☐ Avoid combination of certain drugs
- Narcotics with psychotropics
- More than one psychotropic
Notes:

Appendix G

Sample Home Fall Prevention Safety Checklist

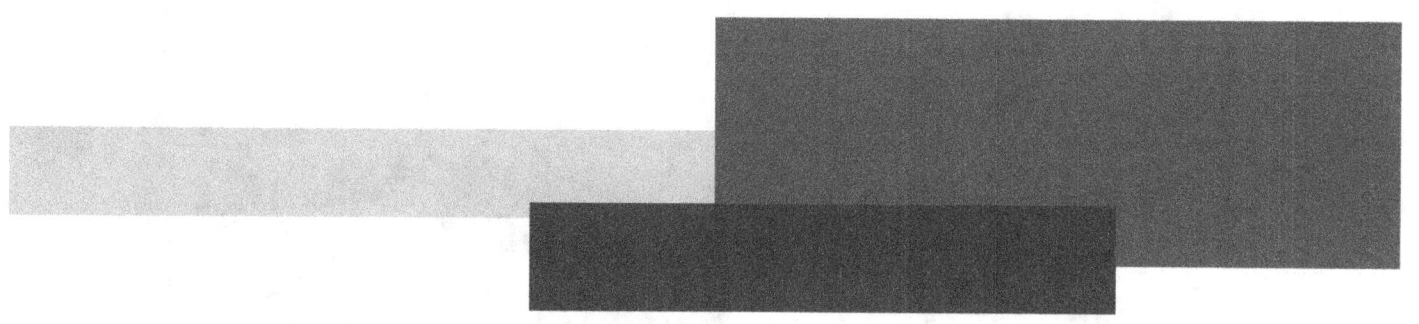

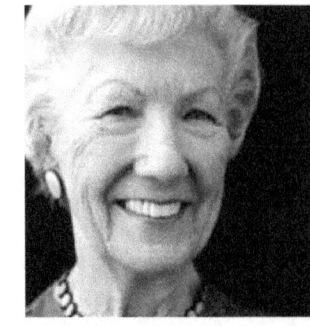
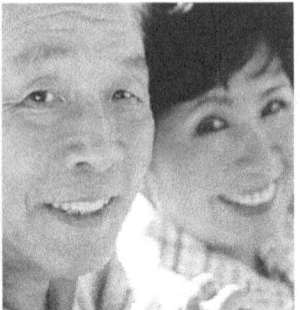

This checklist is based on the original version printed by the Centers for Disease Control and Prevention. Support for this version was provided by MetLife Foundation.

2005

Check for Safety

CDC FOUNDATION

MetLife Foundation

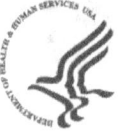 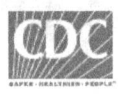

Department of Health and Human Services
Centers for Disease Control and Prevention

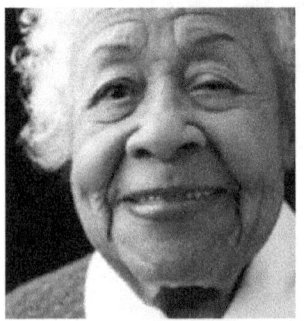

A Home Fall Prevention Checklist for Older Adults

    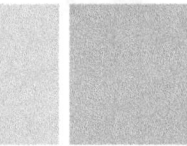  

For more information, contact:
Centers for Disease Control and Prevention
770-488-1506
www.cdc.gov/injury

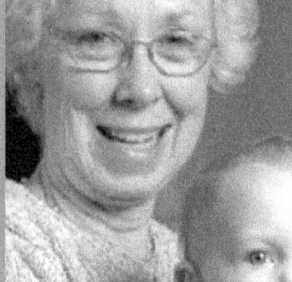

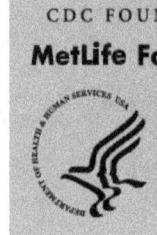
CDC FOUNDATION

MetLife Foundation

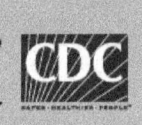

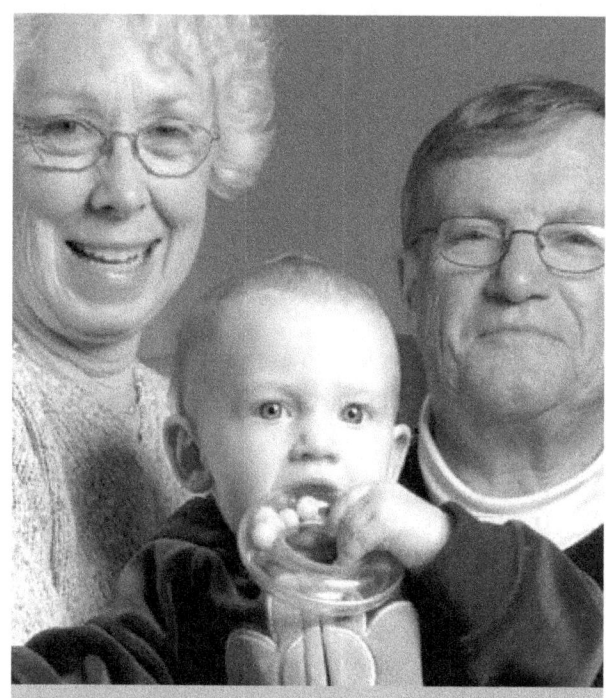

"Making changes in our home to prevent falls is good for us and for our granddaughter when she comes to visit."

FALLS AT HOME

Each year, thousands of older Americans fall at home. Many of them are seriously injured, and some are disabled. In 2002, more than 12,800 people over age 65 died and 1.6 million were treated in emergency departments because of falls.

Falls are often due to hazards that are easy to overlook but easy to fix. This checklist will help you find and fix those hazards in your home.

The checklist asks about hazards found in each room of your home. For each hazard, the checklist tells you how to fix the problem. At the end of the checklist, you'll find other tips for preventing falls.

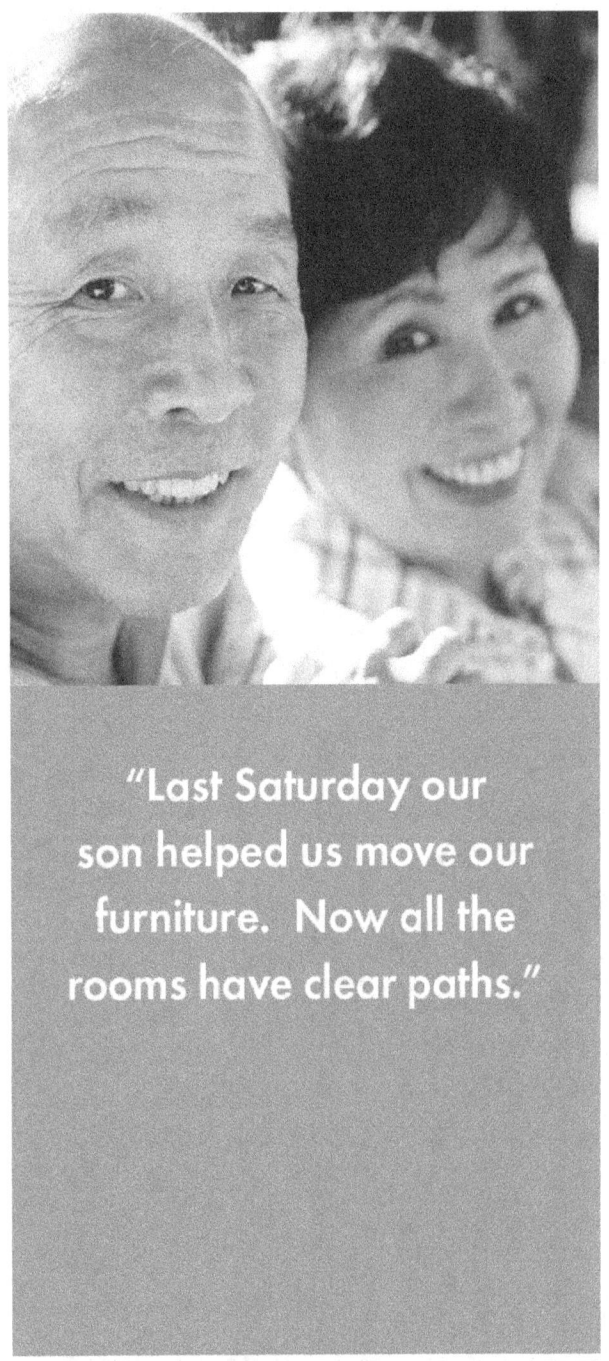

"Last Saturday our son helped us move our furniture. Now all the rooms have clear paths."

FLOORS: Look at the floor in each room.

Q: When you walk through a room, do you have to walk around furniture?

☐ Ask someone to move the furniture so your path is clear.

Q: Do you have throw rugs on the floor?

☐ Remove the rugs or use double-sided tape or a non-slip backing so the rugs won't slip.

Q: Are there papers, books, towels, shoes, magazines, boxes, blankets, or other objects on the floor?

☐ Pick up things that are on the floor. Always keep objects off the floor.

Q: Do you have to walk over or around wires or cords (like lamp, telephone, or extension cords)?

☐ Coil or tape cords and wires next to the wall so you can't trip over them. If needed, have an electrician put in another outlet.

STAIRS AND STEPS:
Look at the stairs you use
both inside and outside
your home.

Q: Are there papers, shoes, books, or other objects on the stairs?

☐ Pick up things on the stairs. Always keep objects off stairs.

Q: Are some steps broken or uneven?

☐ Fix loose or uneven steps.

Q: Are you missing a light over the stairway?

☐ Have an electrician put in an overhead light at the top and bottom of the stairs.

Q: Do you have only one light switch for your stairs (only at the top or at the bottom of the stairs)?

☐ Have an electrician put in a light switch at the top and bottom of the stairs. You can get light switches that glow.

Q: Has the stairway light bulb burned out?

☐ Have a friend or family member change the light bulb.

Q: Is the carpet on the steps loose or torn?

☐ Make sure the carpet is firmly attached to every step, or remove the carpet and attach non-slip rubber treads to the stairs.

Q: Are the handrails loose or broken? Is there a handrail on only one side of the stairs?

☐ Fix loose handrails or put in new ones. Make sure handrails are on both sides of the stairs and are as long as the stairs.

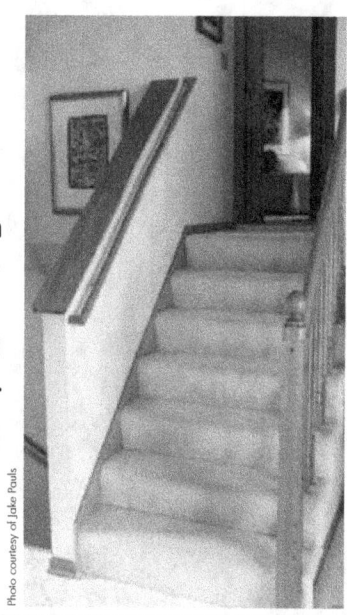

Photo courtesy of Jake Pauls

KITCHEN: Look at your kitchen and eating area.

Q: Are the things you use often on high shelves?

☐ Move items in your cabinets. Keep things you use often on the lower shelves (about waist level).

Q: Is your step stool unsteady?

☐ If you must use a step stool, get one with a bar to hold on to. Never use a chair as a step stool.

BATHROOMS: Look at all your bathrooms.

Q: Is the tub or shower floor slippery?

☐ Put a non-slip rubber mat or self-stick strips on the floor of the tub or shower.

Q: Do you need some support when you get in and out of the tub or up from the toilet?

☐ Have a carpenter put grab bars inside the tub and next to the toilet.

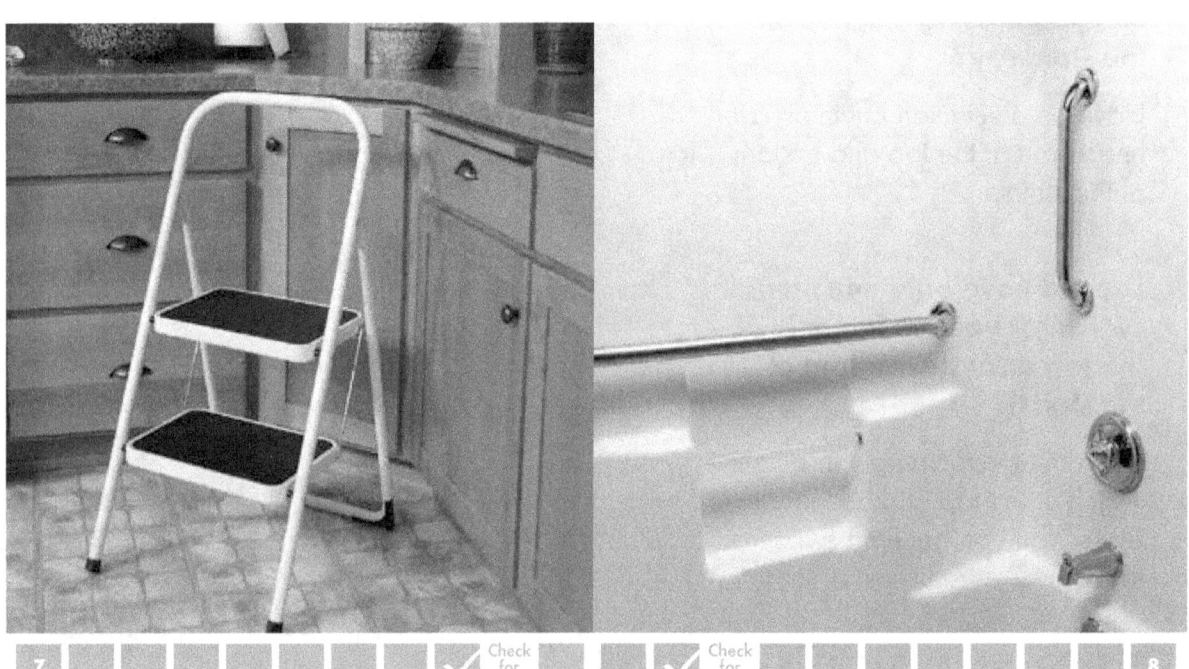

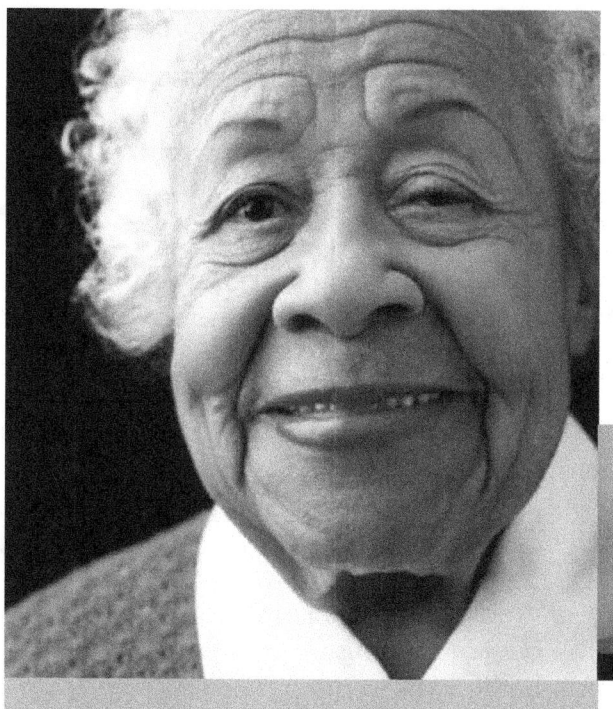

BEDROOMS: Look at all your bedrooms.

Q: **Is the light near the bed hard to reach?**

☐ Place a lamp close to the bed where it's easy to reach.

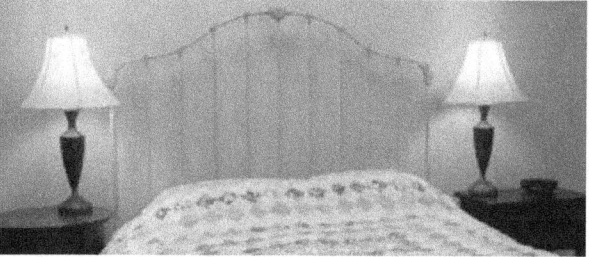

"I put a lamp on each side of my bed. Now it's easy to find the light if I wake up at night."

Q: **Is the path from your bed to the bathroom dark?**

☐ Put in a night-light so you can see where you're walking. Some night-lights go on by themselves after dark.

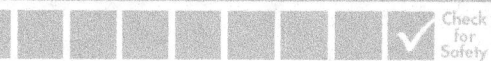

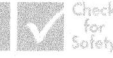

9 · Check for Safety · Check for Safety · 10

83

Other Things You Can Do to Prevent Falls

☐ Exercise regularly. Exercise makes you stronger and improves your balance and coordination.

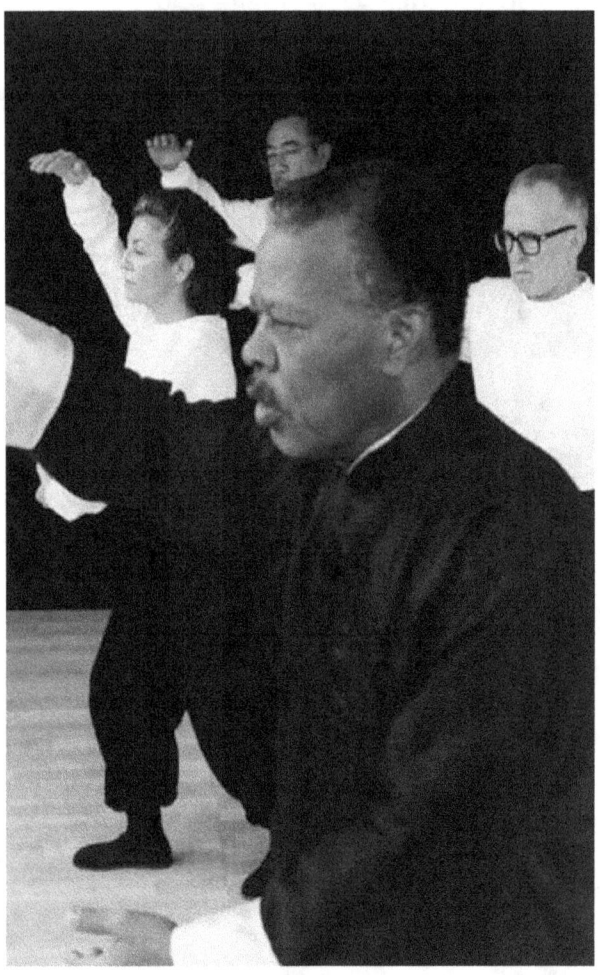

☐ Have your doctor or pharmacist look at all the medicines you take, even over-the-counter medicines. Some medicines can make you sleepy or dizzy.

☐ Have your vision checked at least once a year by an eye doctor. Poor vision can increase your risk of falling.

☐ Get up slowly after you sit or lie down.

☐ Wear shoes both inside and outside the house. Avoid going barefoot or wearing slippers.

☐ Improve the lighting in your home. Put in brighter light bulbs. Florescent bulbs are bright and cost less to use.

☐ It's safest to have uniform lighting in a room. Add lighting to dark areas. Hang lightweight curtains or shades to reduce glare.

☐ Paint a contrasting color on the top edge of all steps so you can see the stairs better. For example, use a light color paint on dark wood.

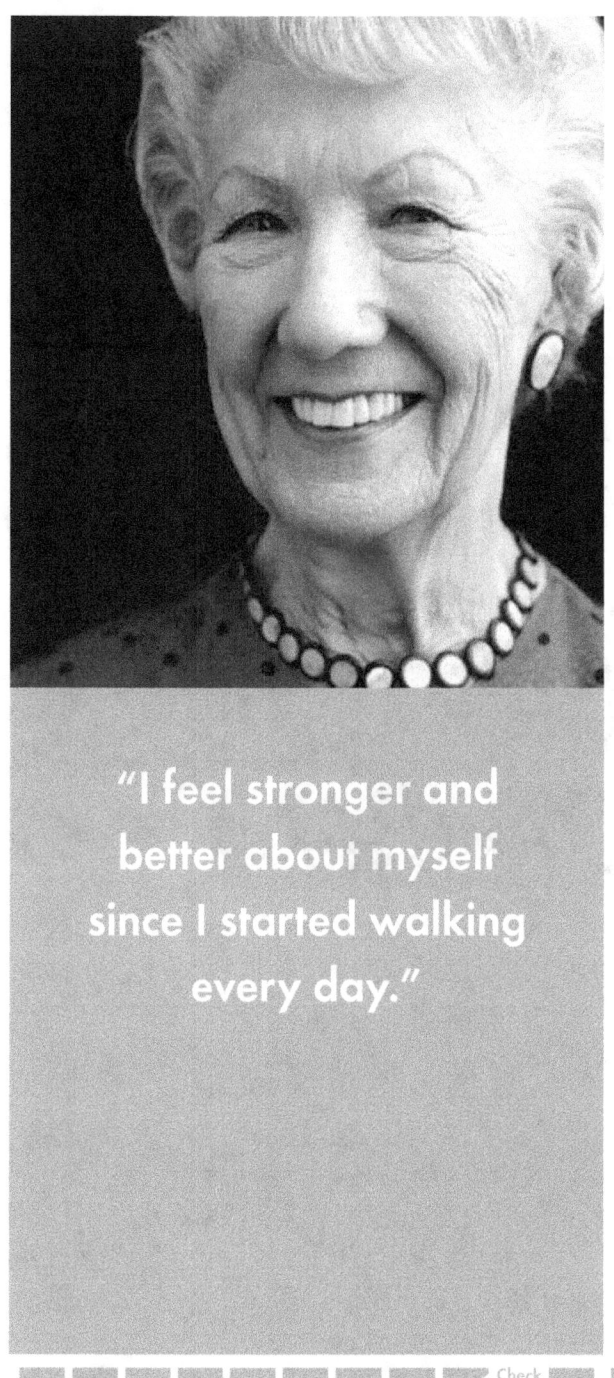

"I feel stronger and better about myself since I started walking every day."

Other Safety Tips

☐ Keep emergency numbers in large print near each phone.

☐ Put a phone near the floor in case you fall and can't get up.

☐ Think about wearing an alarm device that will bring help in case you fall and can't get up.

Appendix H

Sample Program
Evaluation Tool

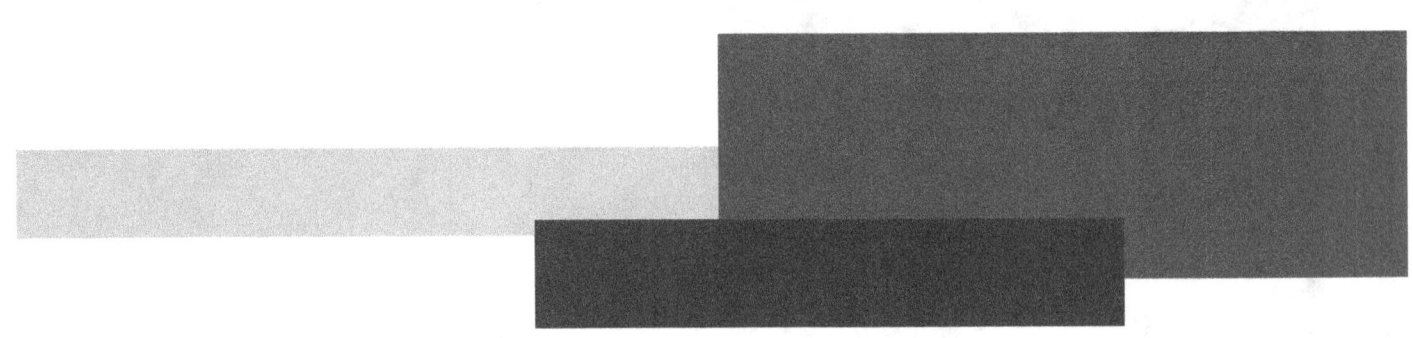

Appendix H - Program Evaluation Checklist

Program Evaluation Checklist

This is a checklist of tasks that organizations developing fall prevention programs can follow to make sure no evaluation steps are omitted during program development, operation, and completion.

1. Program Development
As soon as you or someone in your organization has the idea for a fall prevention program, begin evaluation.

☐ Investigate to make sure an effective program similar to the one you envision does not already exist in your community.

☐ If a similar program does exist *and* if it is fully meeting the needs of your proposed target population, modify your ideas for the program so that you can fill a need that is not being met.

☐ Decide where you will seek financial support.

☐ Find out which federal, state, or local government agencies give grants for the type of program you envision.

☐ Find out which businesses and community groups are likely to support your goals and provide funds to achieve them.

☐ Decide where you will seek non-financial support.

☐ Find out which federal, state, or local government agencies provide technical assistance for the type of program you envision.

☐ Find out which businesses and community groups support your goals and are likely to provide technical assistance, staff, or other non-financial support.

☐ Develop an outline of a plan for your fall prevention program. Include in the outline the methods you will use to provide the program service to participants and the methods you will use to evaluate your program's impact and outcome.

☐ Evaluate the outline. For example, conduct personal interviews or focus groups with a small number of the people you will try to reach with your fall prevention program. Consult people who have experience with programs similar to the one you envision, and ask them to review your plan. Modify your plan on the basis of evaluation results.

Appendix H - Program Evaluation Checklist

☐ Develop a plan to enlist financial and non-financial support from all the agencies, businesses, and community organizations you have decided are likely sources of support. Use the outline of your plan for the injury prevention program to demonstrate your commitment, expertise, and research.

☐ Evaluate the plan for obtaining support. For example, conduct personal interviews with business leaders in your community. Modify your plan on the basis of evaluation results.

☐ Put your plan for obtaining support into action.

☐ Keep track of all contacts you make with potential supporters.

☐ If unexpected problems arise while you are seeking support, re-evaluate your plan or the aspect of your plan that seems to be the source of the problem. For example, if businesses are contributing much less than you had good reason to expect, then seek feedback from businesses that are contributing and those that are not. Or if you did not receive grant funds for which you believed you were qualified, contact the funding agency to find out why your proposal was rejected. Modify your plan according to your re-evaluation results, and continue seeking support.

☐ When you have enough support for your program, expand on the outline of your plan for the fall prevention program. Include in the design a mechanism for evaluating the program's impact and outcome.

☐ Evaluate your program's procedures, materials, and activities. For example, conduct focus groups within your target population. Modify the plan on the basis of evaluation results.

☐ Develop forms to keep track of program participants, program supporters, and all contacts with participants, supporters, or other people outside the program.

☐ Measure the target population's knowledge, attitudes, beliefs, and behaviors that relate to your program goals. The results are your baseline measurements.

Appendix H - Program Evaluation Checklist

2. Program Operation

Put your program into operation.

☐ Track all program-related contacts (participants, supporters, or others). Track all items either distributed to or collected from participants.

☐ As soon as the program has completed its first encounter with the target population, assess any changes in program participants' knowledge, attitudes, beliefs, and (if appropriate) behaviors.

☐ Continue tracking and assessing program-related changes in participants throughout the life of the program. Keep meticulous records.

☐ If unexpected problems arise while the program is in operation, re-evaluate (using qualitative methods) to find the cause and solution. For example, your records might show that not as many people as expected are responding to your program's message, or your assessment of program participants might show that their knowledge is not increasing. Modify the program on the basis of evaluation results.

☐ Evaluate ongoing programs (e.g., exercise and education classes) at suitable intervals to see how well the program is meeting its goal of reducing fall related morbidity and mortality.

3. Program Completion

☐ Use the data you have collected throughout the program to evaluate how well the program met its goals: to increase behaviors that prevent falls and, consequently, to reduce the rate of falls and fall injuries.

☐ Use the results of this evaluation to justify continued funding and support for your program.

☐ If appropriate, publish the results of your program in a scientific journal.

This tool was based on guidelines from the Demonstrating Your Program's Worth, A Primer on Evaluation for Programs to Prevent Unintentional Injury (CDC NCIPC, 2000), a book designed to help program staff understand the processes involved in planning, designing, and implementing evaluation of programs to prevent unintentional injuries.

www.cdc.gov/ncipc/pub-res/demonstr.htm

Appendix I
Sample Pitch Letter

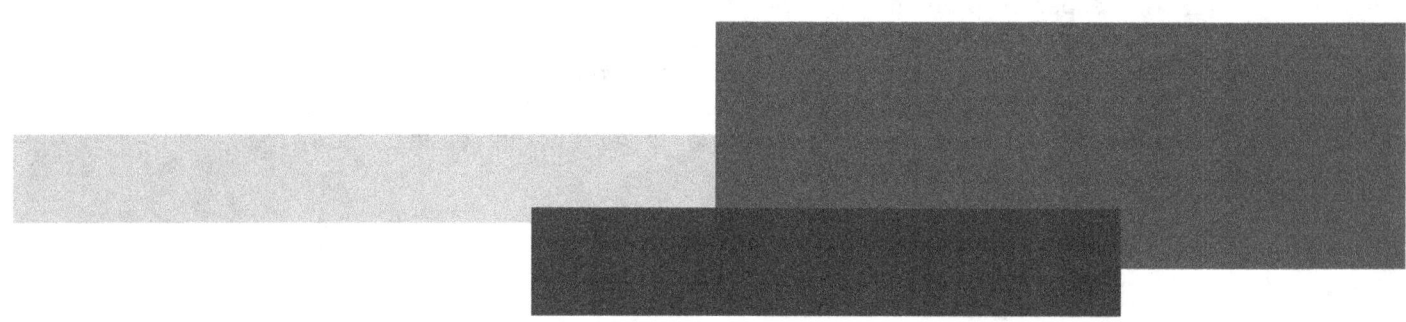

Appendix I - Sample Letter to Health Care Referral Source

[Title]
[Name of organization]
[Address]

Dear [Name]:
Our organization needs your help in preventing falls among older adults—the leading cause of injury deaths and nonfatal injuries for persons aged 65 and older. We are offering a [free/low-cost] fall prevention [exercise class, counseling, home visits, etc.] to individuals whose current health status places them at increased risk of falling. Please recommend our service, described in more detail below, to your patients who would benefit from it.

Our program is [name and description of program; program details. For example:

"Stay Safe, Stay Active," an evidence-based exercise program for older adults at risk of falling due to lower limb weakness, poor balance, slow reaction time, or a combination of these symptoms. We will hold 37 weekly classes of moderate exercise, led by a trained fitness instructor, beginning March 1, from 9 to 10 a.m., at the YMCA at 321 Main Street, Anytown. We will also provide participants with fall prevention strategies and exercises to do at home. Participants will improve their balance and coordination, muscle strength, reaction time, and aerobic capacity while reducing their likelihood of falling or being injured in a fall.]

The Centers for Disease Control and Prevention has identified this intervention as effective in preventing falls.

More than one-third of people aged 65 and older fall each year. Help your patients maintain their health and independence by learning how to avoid falls. Please call me at [telephone number] if you would like further information. [Recommended step: (Program) fliers to distribute to high-risk patients are available.]

Sincerely,

[Your name and title]

Appendix J
Key Points

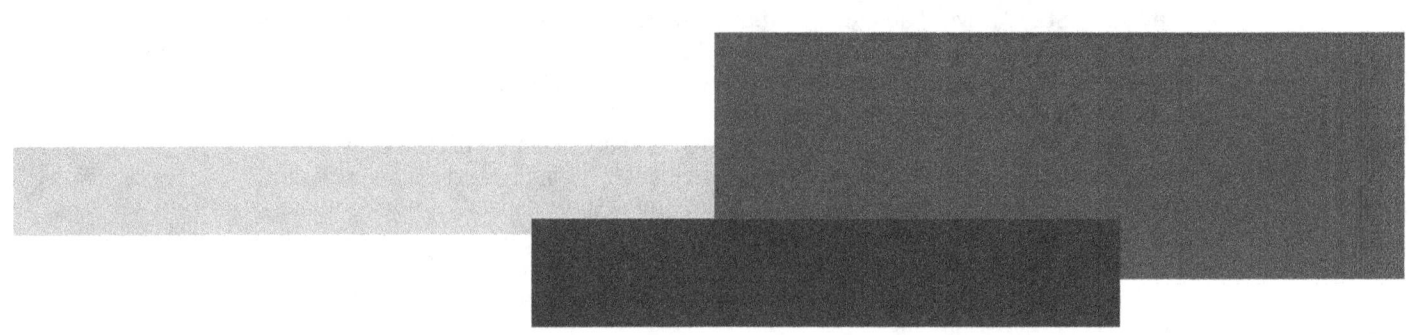

Appendix J - Key Points Regarding Falls Among Older Adults

Health Consequences of Falls (age 65+)

- Falls are a major threat to the health and independence of older adults.

- Each year in the United States, nearly one-third of older adults experience a fall.

- Falls are the leading cause of injury deaths and the most common cause of nonfatal injuries and hospital admissions for persons aged 65 and older.

- In 2004, more than 14,900 people aged 65 or older died of a fall-related injury. Another 1.85 million were treated in emergency departments for nonfatal injuries related to falls.

- About one out of ten falls among older adults results in a serious injury (such as a hip fracture or head injury) that requires hospitalization.

- In 2004, one adult died from a fall every 35 minutes. Every hour, 211 older adults were treated in emergency rooms for fall-related injuries.

- In 2000, direct medical costs totaled $179 million for fatal falls and $19 billion for nonfatal fall injuries.

- In [your state/community], falls account for [X percentage] of emergency room visits by people aged 65 or older.

- In [your state/community], falls account for [X percentage] of hospital admissions for injuries among older adults.

- In [your state/community], falls account for [X percentage] of deaths among older adults.

  (Contact your local hospital, agency on aging or county or state health department for statistics on fall-related injuries and deaths.)

Biological risk factors
- ✓ Mobility problems due to muscle weakness or balance problems
- ✓ Chronic health conditions such as arthritis and stroke
- ✓ Vision changes and vision loss
- ✓ Loss of sensation in feet

Behavioral risk factors
- ✓ Inactivity
- ✓ Medication side effects and/or interactions
- ✓ Alcohol use

Environmental risk factors
- ✓ Home and environmental hazards (clutter, poor lighting, etc.)
- ✓ Incorrect size, type, or use of assistive devices (walkers, canes, crutches, etc.)
- ✓ Poorly designed public spaces

Appendix K

Sustainability Plan Template

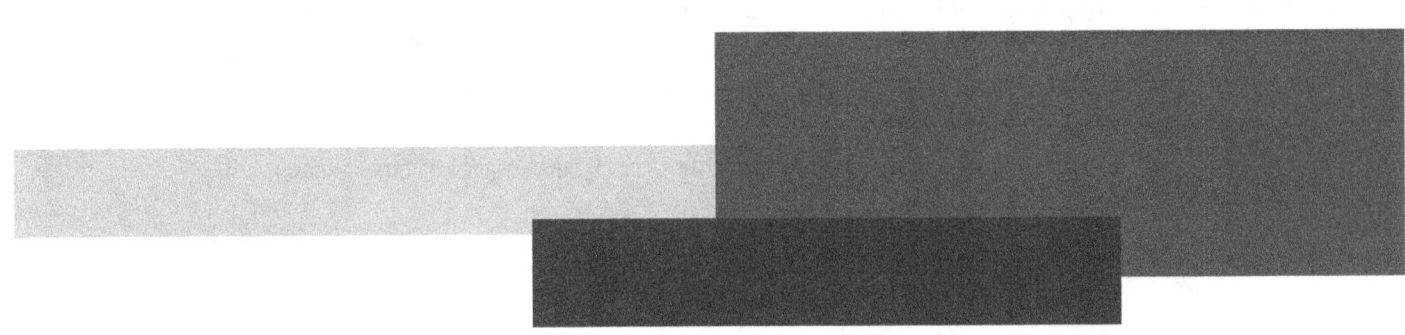

Appendix K - Template for Developing a SUSTAINABILITY PLAN

****
Sustainability Plan for {Your Program Name}

Program Summary
Describe what your program offers, who it serves, when it operates, how it is funded and who your community partners are.

Vision
What is the program's vision? What results do you hope to achieve, and what are the activities that will lead to the desired results? Who will benefit?

Collaborators
Who are your partners? What are their roles, what resources do they contribute, and how do they figure in your sustainability plan?

Advocates
Who are your supporters? What are their goals and how are they providing help?

Current Funding Sources
Who is providing funding for your program? How long will they continue their contributions?

New Potential Funding Sources
List possible funders who could provide additional support. Describe a plan to approach potential funders. Get additional referrals for both public and private funders through partners.

Program Offerings
State specifically how the program addresses the needs of the older adult participants, partners, and the community. Remember to include how your program incorporates effective intervention components to achieve its goals.

Management
Include how you are managing your program's fiscal resources. Describe staffing and information management.

Evaluation
Describe how you will collect information to show results. What tools will you use to collect data? State how you will adapt the program to ensure you are maintaining the vision and meeting your objectives.